Achilles Tendon

Guest Editor

G. ANDREW MURPHY, MD

FOOT AND ANKLE CLINICS

www.foot.theclinics.com

Consulting Editor
MARK S. MYERSON, MD

December 2009 • Volume 14 • Number 4

SAUNDERS an imprint of ELSEVIER, Inc.

W.B. SAUNDERS COMPANY
A Division of Elsevier Inc.

1600 John F. Kennedy Blvd. ● Suite 1800 ● Philadelphia, PA 19103-2899

http://www.theclinics.com

FOOT AND ANKLE CLINICS Volume 14, Number 4
December 2009 ISSN 1083-7515, ISBN-10: 1-4377-1218-5, ISBN-13: 978-1-4377-1218-6

Editor: Debora Dellapena

Foot and Ankle Clinics (ISSN 1083-7515) is published quarterly by Elsevier, Inc., 360 Park Avenue South, New York, NY 10010-1710. Months of issue are March, June, September, and December. Periodicals postage paid at New York, NY, and additional mailing offices. Subscription price per year is $253.00 (US individuals), $340.00 (US institutions), $128.00 (US students), $283.00 (Canadian individuals), $402.00 (Canadian institutions), $175.00 (Canadian students), $364.00 (foreign individuals), $402.00 (foreign institutions), and $175.00 (foreign students). To receive student/resident rate, orders must be accompanied by name of affiliated institution, date of term, and the *signature* of program/residency coordinator on institution letterhead. Orders will be billed at individual rate until proof of status is received. Foreign air speed delivery is included in all *Clinics* subscription prices. All prices are subject to change without notice. **POSTMASTER:** Send address changes to *Foot and Ankle Clinics*, Elsevier Health Sciences Division, Subscription Customer Service, 3251 Riverport Lane, Maryland Heights, MO 63043. **Customer Service: 1-800-654-2452 (US and Canada). From outside of the United States and Canada, call 314-447-8871. Fax: 314-417-8029. E-mail: JournalsCustomerService-usa@ elsevier.com (for print support); JournalsOnlineSupport-usa@elsevier.com (for online support).**

Reprints. For copies of 100 or more, of articles in this publication, please contact the Commercial Reprints Department, Elsevier Inc., 360 Park Avenue South, New York, NY 10010-1710. Tel.: 212-633-3812; Fax: 212-462-1935; E-mail: reprints@elsevier.com.

Printed and bound by CPI Group (UK) Ltd, Croydon, CR0 4YY

Transferred to Digital Print 2011

Contributors

CONSULTING EDITOR

MARK S. MYERSON, MD
Director, Institute for Foot and Ankle Reconstruction, Mercy Medical Center, Baltimore, Maryland

GUEST EDITOR

G. ANDREW MURPHY, MD
Assistant Professor, Department of Orthopaedic Surgery, Campbell Clinic, University of Tennessee, Memphis, Tennessee

AUTHORS

FREDERICK M. AZAR, MD
Professor, Department of Orthopaedic Surgery, Campbell Clinic, University of Tennessee, Memphis, Tennessee

JOHN T. CAMPBELL, MD
Surgeon, Institute for Foot and Ankle Reconstruction, Mercy Medical Center, Faculty, Orthopaedic Foot and Ankle Fellowship Program, Baltimore, Maryland

MARK M. CASILLAS, MD
Clinical Associate Professor, Department of Orthopaedic Surgery, The University of Texas Health Science Center at San Antonio; The Foot and Ankle Center of South Texas, San Antonio, Texas

LAN CHEN, MD
Post-Doctoral Graduate Fellow, Department of Orthopaedic Surgery, Columbia University Medical Center, New York, New York

JOSÉ CARLOS COHEN, MD
Chief of Foot and Ankle Service, Department of Orthopaedic Surgery, National University Hospital of Rio de Janeiro UFRJ-Brazil; Member of the American Orthopaedic Foot and Ankle Society (AOFAS) and the Brazilian Society of Foot Surgery (ABTPE), Rio de Janeiro, Brazil

MARK S. DAVIES, FRCS (Tr & Orth)
Consultant Orthopaedic Surgeon and Clinical Director, The London Foot and Ankle Centre, The Hospital of St. John and St. Elizabeth, London, United Kingdom

BRYAN D. DEN HARTOG, MD
Assistant Clinical Professor, Sanford School of Medicine, University of South Dakota; Black Hills Orthopaedic and Spine Center, Rapid City, South Dakota

JUSTIN GREISBERG, MD
Assistant Professor, Department of Orthopaedic Surgery, Columbia University Medical Center, New York, New York

SUSAN N. ISHIKAWA, MD
Assistant Professor and Foot and Ankle Fellowship Director, Department of Orthopaedics, Campbell Clinic, University of Tennessee, Memphis, Tennessee

ANISH R. KADAKIA, MD
Assistant Professor, Department of Orthopaedic Surgery, Division of Foot and Ankle Surgery, University of Michigan, Ann Arbor, Michigan

JASON E. LAKE, MD
Department of Orthopaedics, Campbell Clinic, University of Tennessee, Memphis, Tennessee

JOHNNY L. LIN, MD
Assistant Professor, Department of Orthopaedic Surgery, Rush University Medical Center, Chicago, Illinois

ANDY MOLLOY, FRCS (Tr & Orth)
Consultant Orthopaedic Surgeon, University Hospital Aintree, Liverpool, United Kingdom

G. ANDREW MURPHY, MD
Assistant Professor, Department of Orthopaedic Surgery, Campbell Clinic, University of Tennessee, Memphis, Tennessee

THOMAS G. PADANILAM, MD
Assistant Clinical Professor, University of Toledo; Toledo Orthopaedic Surgeons, Toledo, Ohio

SETH ROSENZWEIG, MD
Dauterive Orthopaedics and Sports Medicine, New Iberia, Louisiana

BRIAN SABB, DO
Clinical Lecturer, Department of Radiology, University of Michigan, Ann Arbor, Michigan

MATTHEW SOLAN, FRCS (Tr & Orth)
Consultant Orthopaedic Surgeon, The London Foot and Ankle Centre, The Hospital of St. John and St. Elizabeth, London; Consultant Orthopaedic Surgeon, Department of Orthopaedic Surgery, Royal Surrey County Hospital and Consultant Orthopaedic Surgeon, Surrey Foot and Ankle Clinic, Guildford Nuffield Hospital, Guildford, Surrey, United Kingdom

ADAM C. STROM
Dartmouth College, Hanover, New Hampshire

GISELLE TAN, MD
Senior Resident, Department of Orthopaedic Surgery, University of Michigan, Ann Arbor, Michigan

EDWARD V. WOOD, FRCS (Tr & Orth)
Consultant Orthopaedic Surgeon, Countess of Chester Hospital, Chester, Cheshire, United Kingdom

Contents

The complexity of its anatomy coupled with the biomechanics of the Achilles tendon may explain the frequency of injury to this structure. Its unique characteristic of the muscle crossing three joints (knee, ankle, and subtalar joints) makes it more susceptible to injury than muscles that span a single joint. A better understanding of the contributing pathologic conditions associated with functional shortening of the gastroc-soleus complex and its effects on the normal biomechanics of the foot and ankle may improve the treatment of the many and varied pathologies that occur within the tendon itself and the associated abnormalities that occur with a tight Achilles tendon.

Contracture of the gastrocnemius-soleus complex with equinus deformity is a common hindfoot condition. In children, it is frequently associated with neuromuscular conditions such as cerebral palsy. In the adult population, it is linked to numerous pathologies such as adult-acquired flatfoot, diabetic neuropathic ulcers, and plantar fasciitis. With the medial column reduced, failure to achieve 10° of passive ankle dorsiflexion with the knee flexed and extended suggests a contracture. This article reviews the anatomical and evolutionary basis for human foot structure, implications of tight gastrocnemius, and specific disease states. Operative releases for lengthening, including proximal gastrocnemius recession, tendo-Achilles lengthening, and endoscopic recession, are detailed.

Insertional Achilles tendinopathy can be a painful debilitating condition that should initially be treated non-operatively. If pain becomes chronic and debilitating, despite appropriate conservative treatment, debridement of the diseased portion of the Achilles tendon and removal of the impinging calcaneal prominence and transfer of the flexor hallucis longus through a single incision can be a reliable pain relieving procedure with relatively high patient satisfaction.

Noninsertional Achilles tendinitis is a distinct clinical entity, frequently characterized by swelling, pain, and lower limb dysfunction. This condition can be frustrating to treat, for the patient and the physician alike, as reflected in the various treatments, both conservative and surgical, that have been described. Although many patients with Achilles tendinitis can be successfully treated with nonoperative methods, persistent symptoms require surgical treatment, such as tenotomy, debridement, or repair.

Achilles tendinopathy is a painful condition that occurs commonly in both active and inactive individuals. It seems that this condition is painful as a result of ingrowth of neural structures and neovessels leading to poor healing, rather than from inflammatory mediators. Traditional conservative measures are often successful. There is a subset of patients who fail to respond to these measures, however, and this has led to the investigation of newer conservative techniques. This article provides a review of many of the emerging techniques in the treatment of Achilles tendinopathy.

Incidence of Achilles tendon injury has increased as people continue to be active in their later years. Although acute rupture of the Achilles tendon is most commonly diagnosed using history and physical examination, improvements in magnetic resonance and ultrasound imaging have led to their routine use in evaluating these injuries. Non-operative versus operative management of acute Achilles tendon ruptures has been the subject of much controversy in the current literature, especially in light of non-operative treatment with functional bracing. This article highlights the current controversy and outlines the rationale for nonsurgical treatment of acute Achilles tendon ruptures.

This article reviews minimal incision techniques in the treatment of acutely ruptured Achilles tendon and the results that can be anticipated from these methods. However, lack of robust prospective randomized studies on the treatment of Achilles tendon rupture makes it impossible to draw conclusions on optimal treatment strategies. The bulk of the evidence available suggests that surgical repair reduces rerupture rates compared with non-operatively treated tendon ruptures. Surgery does have potential complications, but as outlined in the article, using a mini-open or percutaneous technique of repair might result in highly satisfactory outcomes with acceptably low complication rates.

operative techniques. These include tendon rerupture, sural nerve morbidity, wound healing problems, changes in tendon morphology, venous thromboembolism, elongation of the tendon, complex regional pain syndrome, and compartment syndrome. This article delineates the incidence for each of these complications, with differing techniques, methods of avoiding these complications and treatment methods if they occur.

Acute injuries of the Achilles tendon are common among athletes and non-athletes alike. Injuries of other posterior calf muscles are far less common but should be considered in the differential, to ensure proper diagnosis and treatment of patients with calf injuries. This article focuses on these calf injuries, including injuries of the gastrocnemius, plantaris, soleus, and flexor hallucis longus, which may occasionally be mistaken for Achilles tendon disorders.

The operative management of acute Achilles tendon rupture marks the beginning of a comprehensive rehabilitation program. The goals of the rehabilitation program start with the reduction of pain and swelling and the recovery of ankle motion and power. They conclude with the restoration of coordinated activity and safe return to athletic activity. The rehabilitation protocol is directed by the injury and the quality of the repair, along with the patient's age, medical and social history, and athletic inclination. The protocol is dynamic and responsive to changing clinical findings.

THE CLINICS ARE NOW AVAILABLE ONLINE!

Access your subscription at:
www.theclinics.com

FORTHCOMING ISSUES

March 2010
Diabetic Foot and Ankle Trauma Related to Recent International Conflicts
Eric Bluman, MD and James R. Ficke, MD, Guest Editors

June 2010
The Pediatric Foot and Ankle
B. Sullivan, MD, Guest Editor

December 2010
Infection, Ischemia & Amputation
Michael S. Pinzur, MD, Guest Editor

January 2011
Dermatologic Conditions in Foot and Ankle
Nuart De Maller, MD, Guest Editor

RECENT ISSUES

September 2009
Correction of Multiplanar Deformity of the Foot and Ankle
Anish R. Kadakia, MD, Guest Editor

June 2009
Complex Injuries of the Foot and Ankle in Sport
Dawid A. Porter, MD, PhD, Guest Editor

March 2009
The Hallux
John Campbell, MD, Guest Editor

Foreword

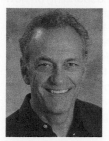

Mark S. Myerson, MD
Consulting Editor

I am certain that the readers are all familiar with the eponymic origin of Achilles to describe the tendon we are so accustomed to treating. There are certainly eponymic uses of injuries, procedures, techniques, and tests, but there are no other anatomic parts of the lower limb that have such significance. Perhaps this is wrapped up in the mythology of the same, or the significance that we attach to this tendon (no pun intended). There are certain treatments of Achilles tendon pathology that I have not changed much in 25 years.

Removal of a postero-superior lateral bone prominence (a Haglund deformity) is one that comes to mind. Management of acute or acute on chronic paratendinitis has not changed much either. There are fortunately or unfortunately so many diverse treatments for Achilles tendon pathology that work reasonably well. We have seen some of these come and go, but the basic issues, with respect to acute or chronic rupture have not changed much.

In my own practice, I have emphasized early range of motion and early weight bearing following treatment of acute ruptures for more than two decades. What I have noted, however, is that there is always some stretching out of the repair during healing and rehabilitation. I used to match the operated and the contralateral limb during surgery so that I could obtain a perfect static resting tension on the operated side. I do not think that this is ideal, and now place the operated foot in far more equinus than I did a decade ago. I have yet to see a limb where the foot is placed in equinus, and return to function, including strength, endurance, and power are compromised. Be careful how you use a boot or cast during the recovery of either acute or chronic ruptures. If your goal is to protect the repair and keep the foot in slight equinus, this must be achieved by placing the foot and not the boot or cast in equinus. If the boot is in equinus, there is a forced leverage on the foot during push off aggravated by the back kneeing that accompanies equinus. This is not the situation if the boot is in neutral and the foot maintained in equinus with pads or wedges.

Have you noticed that regardless of what type of surgical treatment you pursue to manage chronic noninsertional tendinopathy the tendon is generally thicker than before surgery? This seems to be part of the pathologic process of healing. I would

Foot Ankle Clin N Am 14 (2009) xi–xii
doi:10.1016/j.fcl.2009.08.009
1083-7515/09/$ – see front matter © 2009 Elsevier Inc. All rights reserved.

like to think that there are some procedures that work better than others, but I have yet to find one type of reconstruction for chronic noninsertional tendinopathy that is very predictable. All procedures seem to work in the 85% to 90% range, depending on how one defines success. I note that some authors are very optimistic with the use of a transfer of the flexor hallucis longus (FHL) to augment chronic tendinopathy. This is not an unreasonable procedure, but I am always concerned that we are unnecessarily sacrificing the strength of hallucal push off. We all have our "favorite" procedure or technique for management of either insertional or noninsertional tendinopathy, and I do not think that we can be adamant about one or the other. I suspect that in the next decade we will look back at this editorial and recognize that we have come a long way in our understanding of the pathogenesis and treatment of the pathophysiology of Achilles tendinopathy.

Mark S. Myerson, MD
Institute for Foot and Ankle Reconstruction
Mercy Medical Center
301 St. Paul Place
Baltimore, MD 21202, USA

E-mail address:
mark4feet@aol.com (M.S. Myerson)

Preface

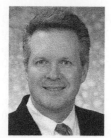

G. Andrew Murphy, MD
Guest Editor

Despite the frequency with which they occur and the many articles written about them, disorders of the Achilles tendon continue to be the subject of controversy. Even the terminology to describe conditions affecting the Achilles tendon is controversial; tendinopathy, tendinosis, tendinitis, tenosynovitis, peritendinitis, and achillodynia, among others, have all been used. The etiology, pathogenesis, and natural history of Achilles disorders remain largely unknown, and there are no definitive criteria to differentiate acute from chronic conditions. Although most acute Achilles tendon injuries occur in athletes involved in sports that require repetitive impact loading, such as jumping or running, approximately 25% of patients with Achilles tendon injuries have no history of athletic involvement, resulting in a diverse patient group requiring individualized treatment considerations. Recommendations for a variety of operative and nonoperative treatment methods often are based on empiric evidence rather than scientific data, and new treatment protocols are continually being developed. There are few prospective, randomized, controlled trials available for a comparison of the different treatments. All of these factors make the treatment of Achilles tendon disorders, ranging from chronic overuse tendinopathy to acute tendon rupture, a challenging problem for orthopedists.

Any discussion of the Achilles tendon should include the indications for and technique of lengthening of the tendon, especially in light of growing enthusiasm for Achilles lengthening for a variety of foot and ankle pathologies. For this comprehensive volume, an article on other posterior calf pathologies is included, because a diagnosis of Achilles pain frequently is, in fact, another problem.

In this issue of *Foot and Ankle Clinics of North America*, several foot and ankle and sports medicine specialists share their experience and expertise in managing these complex disorders and discuss indications, contraindications, techniques, and outcomes of a variety of operative and nonoperative treatment methods. It is hoped

Foot Ankle Clin N Am 14 (2009) xiii–xiv
doi:10.1016/j.fcl.2009.08.010
1083-7515/09/$ – see front matter © 2009 Elsevier Inc. All rights reserved.

foot.theclinics.com

that this information will help answer some of the questions about Achilles tendon disorders and serve as a basis for treatment decision making.

G. Andrew Murphy, MD
Department of Orthopaedic Surgery
Campbell Clinic, University of Tennessee
1211 Union Avenue, Suite 510
Memphis, Tennessee 38104, USA

E-mail address:
gmurp@earthlink.net (G.A. Murphy)

Anatomy and Biomechanical Aspects of the Gastrocsoleus Complex

José Carlos Cohen, MD

KEYWORDS

- Gastrocsoleus complex • Achilles tendon • Biomechanics
- Shortening • Gait

The calcaneal or Achilles tendon is the largest and most powerful tendon in the ankle. At its insertion it is 1.2 to 2.5 cm wide and 5 to 6 mm thick at the ankle level.[1,2] The tendon is formed from the fibers of two muscle units: the gastrocnemius muscle, composed of medial and lateral heads, and the soleus muscle. The medial head of the gastrocnemius muscle arises from behind the medial supracondylar ridge and adductor tubercle on the posterior surface of the femur. The lateral head arises from the lateral surface of the lateral condyle of the femur, proximal and posterior to the lateral epicondyle, and attaches above the knee to the posterior aspect of the medial and lateral femoral condyles. The medial head is broader and thicker than the lateral head. Each of these heads has additional attachments from the posterior capsule of the knee joint and from the oblique popliteal ligament.[3] The gastrocnemius crosses three major joints: (1) knee, (2) ankle, and (3) subtalar. The soleus muscle lies deep to the gastrocnemius muscle and originates from the upper part of the posterior tibia, fibula, and interosseus membrane and crosses only the ankle and subtalar joints. The gastrocnemius is considered a flexor of the knee and ankle and is most effective with the ankle plantar flexed and the knee extended; the soleus muscle is most effective with the ankle plantar flexed and the knee flexed.[4] Both heads of the gastrocnemius are subject to contracture and functional shortening, the pathogenic factors common to many midfoot and forefoot problems. Baudet[5] demonstrated that the medial head of the gastrocnemius is typically tighter than the lateral head and is responsible for most of the dorsiflexion correction obtained with surgical release. The deeper, underlying soleus component rarely is associated with functional shortening.[6]

Foot and Ankle Service, Department of Orthopaedic Surgery, National University Hospital of Rio de Janeiro UFRJ-Brazil, Rua Alberto de Campos 172 apt 101, CEP: 22411-030 Rio de Janeiro UFRJ-Brazil, Brazil
E-mail address: cohenorto@yahoo.com

Foot Ankle Clin N Am 14 (2009) 617–626
doi:10.1016/j.fcl.2009.08.006
1083-7515/09/$ – see front matter © 2009 Elsevier Inc. All rights reserved.

foot.theclinics.com

The main function of the gastrocnemius muscle is propulsion of the body forward during gait, whereas the soleus is a postural muscle that also acts as a peripheral vascular pump. In a cadaver study, Silver and colleagues[7] determined the strength percentages of the muscles around the foot and ankle to define relative strengths of the muscles: the soleus was 30%, the medial head of the gastrocnemius 13.7%, and the lateral head of the gastrocnemius 5.5%, suggesting that the power of plantar flexion resides primarily in the soleus and not in the gastrocnemius.

The soleus muscle has a complex multipennate architecture that often is oversimplified anatomically. In general, two separate compartments, a bipennate anterior compartment and a unipennate posterior compartment, can be identified within the soleus muscle.[8]

In their proximal aspects, both the gastrocnemius and soleus muscles form an aponeurosis, from each of which originates a tendon. These two tendons freely glide independently before they coalesce into the Achilles tendon, approximately 5 to 6 cm proximal to the calcaneal insertion. The tendinous components of these two muscles are variable. The gastrocnemius component is longer (11–26 cm) than that of the soleus (3–11 cm).[3] Morphologically, the aponeurosis differs from the tendon in that there is a marked gradient in thickness, such that it is thicker distally. Further, it has been shown that the width of the aponeurosis increases with muscle contraction and its length-changes during passive conditions exceeds that during muscle contraction.[9] Magnusson and colleagues[9] measured the in vivo strain patterns of the Achilles tendon alone compared with the aponeurosis of the gastrocsoleus and found that strain of the free Achilles tendon was 5.7 times greater than that of the distal aponeurosis. They concluded that the markedly different strain patterns of the free tendon and the aponeurosis suggests that they may have different functional roles during force transmission.

Oriented nearly in the frontal plane, the Achilles tendon is invested by the superficial crural fascia. The tendon is larger at the insertion on the inferior half of the posterior calcaneal surface. Some of the insertional fibers are in continuity with the plantar aponeurosis[10]; however, the number of fibers that connect the Achilles tendon to the plantar fascia decreases with age.[11] Snow and colleagues[12] evaluated the Achilles tendon insertion and its relation to the plantar fascia and found in neonates a thick continuation of fibers of the tendinous insertion into the plantar fascia that gradually diminishes with age until it becomes a connection of superficial fibers in the middle-aged foot. In elderly individuals, there seem to be separate insertions altogether, with periosteum between the Achilles tendon and the plantar fascia.[3] This association allows the plantar fascia and Achilles tendon to function as a unit.

The plantaris muscle arises in close association with the lateral head of the gastrocnemius; it is absent in 7% of individuals. This flat fusiform muscle is followed by a long, slender tendon that courses obliquely downward and medially between the soleus and both heads of gastrocnemius. The tendon lies along the medial border of the Achilles tendon and has variable insertion patterns. Four distinct insertion patterns have been described[1]: type I (47%), a fan-shaped expansion inserting into the medial aspect of the superior calcaneal tuberosity for the insertion of the Achilles tendon; type II (36.5%), an insertion on the calcaneus, 0.5 to 2.5 cm anterior to the medial border of the Achilles tendon; type III (12.5%), a broad insertion investing the dorsal and medial surfaces of the adjacent terminal Achilles tendon; and type IV (4%), an insertion on the medial border of the Achilles tendon 1 to 16 cm proximal to the insertion of the Achilles tendon on the calcaneus.

The retrocalcaneal bursa lies deep and just proximal to the insertion of the Achilles tendon, between the posterior calcaneal tuberosity and the tendon. Anteriorly, it is composed of fibrocartilage; posteriorly it blends with the paratenon and commonly connects to the posterior Achilles tendon. Superficial to the tendon, the pre-Achilles bursa lies between the tendon and the skin. This bursa is composed of synovium and provides lubrication to assist with tendon gliding and to minimize tendon irritation.[13]

At about the level where the soleus contributes fibers to the Achilles tendon, rotation of the tendon begins.[14] Although the rotation of the fibers from the Achilles tendon has been described[1,10,11] as twisting 90 degrees counterclockwise toward the insertion into the calcaneal tuberosity, with the gastrocnemius fibers lying lateral and the soleus fibers lying medial to the insertion point, the degree of rotation of the tendon is variable, ranging between 30 and 150 degrees. The grouping and distribution of this variability were studied by Cummins and colleagues[1] in 100 tendons (**Fig. 1**). In 52% of subjects the posterior contribution to the Achilles tendon at the level of insertion into the calcaneus was two thirds laterally from the gastrocnemius and one third medially from the soleus, which they considered minimal rotation; in 35% the contribution was equally divided between the gastrocnemius and soleus muscles; and in 13% there was a contribution of one third from the gastrocnemius laterally and two thirds from the soleus medially, producing maximal rotation of the fibers. O'Brien[11] noted that some individuals exhibit a double spiral, where the lateral head of the

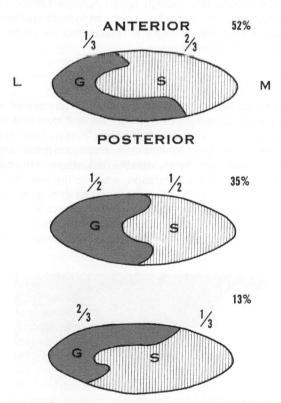

Fig. 1. Degree of rotation of gastrocnemius-to-soleus portion of the calcaneal tendon (left extremity) at the level of insertion into the calcaneus. (*Adapted from* Cummins EJ, Anson JB, Carr WB, et al. The structure of the calcaneal tendon [of Achilles] in relation to orthopedic surgery with additional observations on the plantaris muscle. Surg Gynecol Obstet 1946;83:107–10; with permission.)

gastrocnemius runs from the dorsal side, then comes ventral, and finally turns to the dorsal aspect.

The tendon is rounded proximally and relatively flat distally. Approximately 12 to 15 cm proximal to its insertion, rotation begins and becomes more marked in the distal 5 to 6 cm. This twisting produces stress within the tendon[15] that has been shown to be greatest 2 to 5 cm above the calcaneal insertion, corresponding anatomically with the region of the tendon with the poorest blood supply and the slowest recovery and healing rates, which ultimately becomes the most common site for tendinopathy and rupture.[16,17]

Additionally, it has been postulated that forces of different muscles (medial and lateral heads of the gastrocnemius muscle and the soleus muscle) acting in different directions at the musculotendinous junction of the Achilles tendon may lead to sliding between fibers. These nonhomogenous stresses in different fibers have been suggested as a possible underlying mechanism for tendon injury.[18] In an anatomic study, Arndt and colleagues[18] demonstrated that tensile forces on different triceps surae components resulted in nonhomogenous force distribution across the Achilles tendon, with medial tendon forces significantly higher than lateral when only the medial head of the gastrocnemius was subjected to force. Lateral forces were significantly higher when both heads of gastrocnemius or all three muscles were loaded. This information suggests a possible mechanism through which Achilles tendon injuries, such as tendonitis or tendinosis, may originate. This asymmetric loading of the Achilles tendon caused by its special anatomic structure is responsible for partial ruptures of the Achilles tendon, commonly seen clinically.[14]

BLOOD SUPPLY

The Achilles tendon has no true synovial sheath; it is surrounded by a paratenon, a double-layered sheath composed of an inner, visceral layer and an outer, parietal layer. The visceral layer is connected to the parietal layer by bridges called "mesotenon." The paratenon is a thin, gliding membrane continuous proximally with the fascial envelope of muscle and blending distally with the periosteum of the calcaneus. Nerves and blood vessels run through the paratenon, which is the main blood supply to the middle portion of the tendon (**Fig. 2**). This supply comes through a series of transverse vincula, which function as passageways for blood vessels to reach the tendon. A recurrent branch of the posterior tibial artery supplies the proximal part of the tendon, whereas the distal part is vascularized by the rete arteriosum calcaneare and supplied

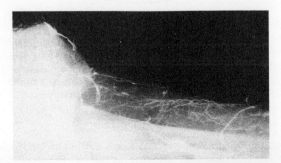

Fig. 2. Radiograph of an injected tendon showing vessels within the paratenon. (*From* Carr AJ, Norris SH. The blood supply of the calcaneal tendon. J Bone Joint Surg Br 1989;71:100–2; with permission.)

by the fibular and posterior tibial arteries.[11] When a paratenon is lined by synovium, it is called a "tenosynovium"; when there is no synovial lining, it is called a "tenovagium." The Achilles tendon has a tenovagium, whereas the other tendons of the ankle have tenosynovium.[19] In addition to these mesotenal vessels, the blood supply to the tendon comes from two other sources: the musculotendinous insertion and the osseous insertion.[3] Carr and Norris[20] demonstrated numerous vessels evenly distributed through the length of the paratenon and, on the anterior surface, vessels running in the mesotenon toward the tendon. When the paratenon was removed, the number of vessels was markedly reduced, although still visible in the muscle and at the osseotendinous junction. Quantitative analysis of the cross-section of the Achilles tendon in relation to the distance from the calcaneus showed in the tendon midsection reductions in both the number and the mean percentage area occupied by blood vessels, comprising a relative zone of hypovascularity within 2 to 6 cm proximal to the calcaneal insertion, in the area of tendon most prone to rupture.[21] Like others tendons, the Achilles has a very low metabolic rate. This feature is important because the Achilles tendon works in constant tension and is more susceptible to ischemia and necrosis caused by the low oxygen intake. This low metabolic rate also slows down the rate of recovery after activity and of healing after injury.[22]

BIOMECHANICS OF THE GASTROSOLEUS COMPLEX DURING GAIT

When the ankle joint moves in a single plane, all the controlling muscles function either as dorsiflexors or plantar flexors. Timing of ankle muscle action is phasic: the plantar flexors consistently are active in stance, and the dorsiflexors are swing-phase muscles. Seven muscles pass posterior to the ankle and serve as plantar flexors.[23] Their actual capacity, however, varies markedly. The soleus and gastrocnemius account for 93% of the theoretical plantar flexor torque, whereas the five perimalleolar muscles provide 7%.[24] The soleus and medial and lateral heads of the gastrocnemius have the advantage of large size and a full calcaneal lever. Among the perimalleolar muscles, the flexor hallucis longus generates the greatest plantar flexor torque.

The range of motion of the ankle joint[23] during a normal gait cycle is plantar flexion to about 7 degrees, which occurs between 0% and 12% of the gait cycle; dorsiflexion to 10 degrees, which occurs between 12% and 48% of the gait cycle; and plantar flexion to 20 degrees, which occurs at 48% to 62% of the gait cycle. The ankle dorsiflexes to neutral during the swing phase.

Under normal circumstances, the anterior compartment of the leg eccentrically contracts at the heel-strike to decelerate the foot as it rolls into foot-flat, whereas the muscles in the posterior compartment relax. From heel-strike to midstance, the gastrocnemius-soleus complex remains inactive, allowing progressive eversion of the subtalar joint. As the hindfoot assumes a valgus position, the axes of the talonavicular and calcaneal-cuboid joints become parallel, unlock, and permit abduction through the transverse tarsal joints.[23] This creates the ideal environment for the shock-absorbing function of the midfoot during midstance. During the late midstance and terminal stance, just before the heel-rise phase of gait, the foot must become a rigid lever arm to propel the body forward. This is accomplished by the locking mechanism that occurs through the midfoot, when the subtalar inversion caused by the contraction of the posterior tibial muscle causes the axes of the talonavicular and calcaneal joints to diverge. This locks the midtarsal joint into relative plantar flexion. The tarsometatarsal joints also are locked by this mechanism. The subtalar inversion shifts the insertion of the Achilles tendon medial to the axis of rotation of the subtalar joint. Such mechanism transforms the foot into a rigid lever, which together with the contraction of the Achilles complex makes the foot capable of propelling the body forward through push-off from the metatarsal heads.[25] The plantar flexion moment of both heads of the gastrocnemius are significantly higher than that of the soleus.[26]

The gastrocsoleus complex is a stance-phase muscle whose activity begins at about 10% of the gait cycle; maximal intensity occurs at 40% and activity ceases at 50% of the gait cycle (**Fig. 3**). The main function of the gastrocsoleus complex is to restrain the forward movement of the tibia over the stance foot. Push-off by the foot during normal steady-state walking is not thought to occur, but it certainly does occur in sporting activities.[27] Biomechanical force analysis has demonstrated that the Achilles tendon is subjected to forces up to 10 times bodyweight during running.[28]

Before quantitative analysis and mechanical modeling, heel-rise was imprecisely perceived as active ankle plantar flexion and referred to as "push-off," which implies propulsion, but this is misleading. Although the ankle plantar flexors are active, they are resisting the external dorsiflexion moment, effectively stabilizing the ankle joint and promoting controlled tibial advancement over the forefoot.[29]

An in vitro study[26] showed that besides the plantar flexion and inversion forces produced by the Achilles tendon, a tensile force applied solely to the lateral head of the gastrocnemius produced an eversion moment at the calcaneus, whereas all other configurations of muscle loading of the triceps surae demonstrated the expected inversion moment. The authors suggested that the inversion-eversion axis of the foot does not pass lateral to the Achilles tendon but through the tendon insertion.

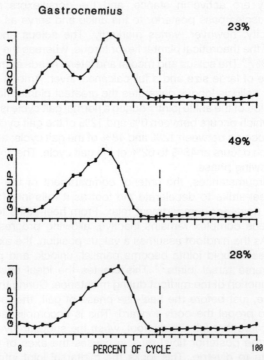

Fig. 3. Patterns of activity of the gastronemius (medial) muscle in three groups of patients. (*From* Wootten ME, Kadaba MP, Cochran GVB. Dynamic electromyography. II. Normal patterns during gait. J Orthop Res 1990;8:259–65; with permission.)

EFFECT OF FUNCTIONAL SHORTENING OF THE GASTROC-SOLEUS COMPLEX

Equinus contracture of the gastroc-soleus complex has been well documented in patients with neurologic or spastic imbalance. Such equinus positioning of the foot occurs not in the Achilles tendon itself, but rather in the muscle bellies of the gastrocmemius or soleus muscles. Isolated soleus contracture in the absence of gastrocnemius pathology has not been documented.[25] More commonly, shortening of the gastroc-soleus complex occurs mainly in two forms: one in which the gastrocnemius muscle alone is affected and another in which both the gastrocnemius and soleus are affected. Although equinus contracture of the ankle usually is caused by systemic disorders, such as neurologic abnormalities, isolated contracture of the gastrocnemius muscle has been reported in otherwise healthy individuals.[30,31] Functional shortening of the gastroc-soleus complex has been implicated as a possible cause of several disorders. The strongest causal relationships have been established between gastroc-soleus contracture and the eventual development of metatarsalgia, neuropathic ulceration, plantar fasciitis, and Charcot midfoot breakdown.[30,32–36]

The tethering action on the posterior aspect of the calcaneus from an unyielding and functionally short Achilles tendon places a plantar-flexion force on the arch of the foot during normal gait,[37] increasing the peak plantar pressures on the forefoot and causing an early heel-rise during the stance phase of the gait cycle.

During the midstance phase of gait, just before heel-lift, the relative length of the gastrocnemius as compared with the length of the tibia becomes significant.[33] At this time, the foot is acting as a base over which the limb and body must rotate in a forward manner. This motion occurs at the ankle and places the gastrocnemius on stretch with the knee in full extension. Even if the gastrocnemius complex cannot expand fully to provide knee and ankle rotation, the rotation still takes place. When mobility cannot occur at the ankle joint, it must be compensated for at some level within the kinetic chain of the lower extremity.

DiGiovanni and Langer[25] emphasized that contracture of the Achilles tendon adversely affects not only the ankle, but also the subtalar joint. Besides the limited ankle dorsiflexion caused by Achilles tendon tightness, contracture of the gastroc-soleus complex exacerbates hindfoot valgus. DiGiovanni and Langer[25] noted that the linkage between ankle and subtalar motion, occurring as dorsiflexion of the ankle coupled with eversion or plantar flexion with inversion of the subtalar joint, suggests that Achilles tendon tightness is not a single-plane deformity, but a multiplane abnormality. During the stance phase of gait, limited dorsiflexion of the ankle (caused by shortening of the gastroc-soleus complex) results in excessive hindfoot pronatory malrotation through the oblique axis of the subtalar joint as a compensatory motion caused by the reactive force from the ground. Eventually, the tight gastroc-soleus complex leads to failure of the medial column of the foot, producing a flatfoot deformity because the subtalar joint is forced into an everted position and can no longer invert during the stance phase of gait. This makes the foot incapable of functioning as a rigid lever arm during push-off and increases repetitive stresses during gait, resulting in attenuation of the plantar medial structures of the foot. Thordarson and colleagues,[38] in a cadaver model, observed that the gastroc-soleus complex was the major factor predisposing to arch flattening in the sagittal plane and an important contributor to forefoot abduction in the transverse plane of the foot. The relationship between malalignment of the subtalar and midtarsal joints with hypermobility has been described[39] as pronation of the rearfoot during the early propulsion phase of gait that causes severe symptomatic hypermobility of the forefoot when the gastroc-soleus complex is shortened. In addition, the first ray becomes hypermobile when the midtarsal joint pronates.[32] This can lead to transverse plane mobility of the first metatarsal with widening of the I-II intermetatarsal angle and consequent hallux valgus and metatarsalgia.

Unfortunately, there is no clear definition of what is considered pathologic in terms of the degree of ankle dorsiflexion that is indicative of shortening of the gastroc-soleus complex. To provide an objective definition of Achilles contracture, DiGiovanni and colleagues[31] used an inability to dorsiflex through the tibiotalar joint, with gastrocnemius equinus present when maximal ankle dorsiflexion was 5 degrees or less with the knee in full extension and Achilles tightness when maximal ankle dorsiflexion was 10 degrees or less with the knee in 90 degrees of flexion.

The usefulness of the Silverskiöld test also has been questioned, with some authors[40,41] stating that it is not possible to clinically differentiate between contractures of the gastrocnemius and the soleus by using this test in a nonanesthetized patient, making it difficult to locate the primary cause of shortening of the gastroc-soleus complex during walking.

Long-term functional shortening of the gastroc-soleus complex, notably the gastrocnemius component, has detrimental effects on patients without neurologic impairment, affecting not only the biomechanics during gait but also predisposing the individual to a number of pathologic conditions.

SUMMARY

The complexity of its anatomy coupled with the biomechanics of the Achilles tendon may explain the frequency of injury to this structure. Its unique characteristic of the muscle crossing three joints (knee, ankle, and subtalar joints) makes it more susceptible to injury than muscles that span a single joint. A better understanding of the contributing pathologic conditions associated with functional shortening of the gastroc-soleus complex and its effects on the normal biomechanics of the foot and ankle may improve the treatment of the many and varied pathologies that occur within the tendon itself and the associated abnormalities that occur with a tight Achilles tendon.

REFERENCES

1. Cummins JE, Anson JB, Carr WB, et al. The structure of the calcaneal tendon (of Achilles) in relation to orthopaedic surgery with additional observations on the plantaris muscle. Surg Gynecol Obstet 1946;83:107.
2. Testut L. Troité d Anatomie Humaine. (Vol. 1). Paris; Doin: 1921. p. 992 [in French].
3. Schepsis AA, Jones H, Hass AL. Achilles tendon disorders in athletes. Am J Sports Med 2002;30(2):287–305.
4. Murphy GA. Disorders of tendons and fascia. In: Canale ST, editor, Campbell's operative orthopaedics, vol. 4, 10th edition. Philadelphia: Mosby; 2003. p. 4224.
5. Baudet B. The tennis leg. Presented at the International Spring Meeting of the French Foot Societies. Tolouse (France); June 9, 2006.
6. Hansen ST Jr. Heel cord injuries. In: Hansen ST, editor. Functional reconstruction of the foot and ankle. Philadelphia: Lippincott Williams & Wilkins; 2000. p. 39–42.
7. Silver RL, De La Garza J, Rang M. The myth of muscle balance: a study of relative strengths and excursions of normal muscles about the foot and ankle. J Bone Joint Surg Br 1985;67(3):432–7.
8. Finni T, Hodgson JA, Lai AM, et al. Mapping of movement in the isometrically contracting human soleus muscle reveals details of its structural and functional complexity. J Appl Physiol 2003;95:2128–33.

9. Magnusson SP, Hansen P, Aagaard P, et al. Differential strain patterns of the human gastrocnemius aponeurosis and free tendon, in vivo. Acta Physiol Scand 2003;177:185–95.

10. Sarrafian SK. Myology. In: Sarrafian SK, editor. Anatomy of the foot and ankle: descriptive topographic functional. Philadelphia: J.B. Lippincott Company; 1983. p. 199–250.

11. O'Brien M. The anatomy of the Achilles tendon. Foot Ankle Clin 2005;10:225–38.

12. Snow SW, Bonne WH, Di Carlo E, et al. Anatomy of the Achilles tendon and plantar fascia in relation to the calcaneus in various age groups. Foot Ankle Int 1995;16:418–21.

13. Title CI, Schon L. Achilles tendon disorders including tendinosis and tears. In: Porter DA, Schon LC, editors. Baxter's the foot and ankle in sport. 2nd edition. Philadelphia: Elsevier; 2008. p. 147–81.

14. Smigielski R. Management of partial tears of the gastro-soleus complex. Clin Sports Med 2008;27:219–29.

15. Henessy MS, Molloy AP, Sturdee SW. Noninsertional Achilles tendinopathy. Foot Ankle Clin 2007;12:617–41.

16. Barfred T. Experimental rupture of Achilles tendon. Acta Orthop Scand 1971;42: 528–43.

17. Benjamin M, Evans EJ, Copp L. The histology of tendon attachment to bone in man. J Anat 1986;149:89–100.

18. Arndt A, Brüggemann GP, Koebke J, et al. Assymetrical loading of the human triceps surae: I. Mediolateral force differences in the Achilles tendon. Foot Ankle Int 1999;20(7):444–9.

19. Smith AM, Sands AK. Achilles tendon problems. In: Di Giovanni C, Greisberg J, editors. Foot and ankle: core knowledge in orthopaedics. Philadelphia: Elsevier; 2007. p. 200–8.

20. Carr AJ, Norris SH. The blood supply of the calcaneal tendon. J Bone Joint Surg Br 1989;71(1):100–1.

21. Curt L, Lindholm A. Vascular distribution in the Achilles tendon: an angiographic and microangiographic study. Acta Chir Scand 1959;116:491–5.

22. Williams JGP. Achilles tendon lesion in sport. Sports Med 1986;3:114–35.

23. Perry J. Ankle foot complex: gait analysis: normal and pathology function. Thorofare (NJ): SLACK, Inc; 1992. p. 51–88.

24. Haxton HA. Absolute muscle force in ankle flexors of man. J Physiol 1944;103: 267–73.

25. DiGiovanni CW, Langer P. The role of isolated gastrocnemius and combined Achilles contractures in the flatfoot. Foot Ankle Clin 2007;12:363–79.

26. Arndt A, Brüggemann GP, Koebke J, et al. Assymetrical loading of the human triceps surae. II. Differences in calcaneal moments. Foot Ankle Int 1999;20(7): 450–5.

27. Hansen ST, Mann RM. Gastrocnemius equinus: is it real, does it affect the foot, and how/when do we treat it [program]? From: American orthopaedic foot and ankle specialty day. San Diego (CA); 2007.

28. Burdett RG. Forces predicted at the ankle during running. Med Sci Sports Exerc 1982;14:308.

29. Davids JR. Normal gait and assessment of gait disorders. In: Morrissy T, Weinstein SL, editors. Lovell and Winter's pediatric orthopaedics. Philadelphia: Lippincott Williams & Wilkins; 2001. p. 131–56.

30. Hill RS. Ankle equines: prevalence and linkage to common foot pathology. J Am Podiatr Med Assoc 1995;85:295–300.

31. DiGiovanni CW, Kuo R, Tejwani N, et al. Isolated gastrocnemius tightness. J Bone Joint Surg Am 2002;84:962–70.
32. Downey MS, Banks AS. Gastrocnemius recession in the treatment of nonspastic ankle equinus: a retrospective study. J Am Podiatr Med Assoc 1989;79:159–74.
33. Sgarlato TE, Morgan J, Shane HS, et al. Tendo Achilles lengthening and its effect on foot disorders. J Am Podiatry Assoc 1975;65:849–71.
34. Kibler WB, Goldberg C, Chandler TJ. Functional biomechanical deficits in running athletes with plantar fasciitis. Am J Sports Med 1991;19:66–71.
35. Armstrong DG, Stracpoole-Shea S, Nguyen H, et al. Lengthening of the Achilles tendon in diabetics patients who are at high risk for ulceration of the foot. J Bone Joint Surg Am 1999;81:535–8.
36. Schon LC, Easley ME, Weinfeld SB. Charcot neuroarthropathy of the foot and ankle. Clin Orthop Relat Res 1998;349:116–31.
37. Grant WP, Sullivan R. Eletron microscopic investigation of the effects of diabetes mellitus on the Achilles tendon. J Foot Ankle Surg 1997;36:272–8.
38. Thodarson DB, Schmotzer H, Chon J, et al. Dynamic support of the human longitudinal arch: a biomechanical evaluation. Clin Orthop Relat Res 1995;316: 165–72.
39. Root ML, Orien WP, Weed JH. Forces acting upon the foot during locomotion. In: Root ML, Orien WP, Weed JH, editors, Normal and abnormal function of the foot, clinical biomechanics, vol. 2. Los Angeles (CA): Clinical Biomechanics Corporation; 1977. p. 165–79.
40. Matjacic Z, Olensek A, Bajd T. Biomechanical characterization and clinical implications of artificially induced toe-walking: differences between pure soleus, pure gastrocnemius, and combination of soleus and gastrocnemius contractures. J Biomech 2006;39(2):255–66.
41. Gage JR. Gait analysis in cerebral palsy. London: MacKeith Press; 1991.

Achilles Lengthening Procedures

Lan Chen, MD, Justin Greisberg, MD*

KEYWORDS

- Gastrocnemius recession • Achilles contracture
- Equinus • Achilles tendon • Lengthening

Contracture of the gastrocnemius-soleus complex, often referred to as an equinus contracture, is a common clinical finding. Severe deformities are obvious and debilitating, such as the contracture following an untreated compartment syndrome of the leg. Other common contractures are seen in adults with neurologic impairment, or following ankle trauma. Neuromuscular problems can lead to equinus contracture in children, especially in cerebral palsy.

THE PROBLEM OF EQUINUS CONTRACTURES

Recently, the existence of isolated gastrocnemius contracture and its clinical impact in the neurologically unaffected population has been explored. This subtle and progressive pathology in neurologically "normal" individuals has been underrecognized.[1] Publications have linked a tight gastrocnemius to adult-acquired flatfoot, metatarsalgia, diabetic forefoot ulceration, and plantar fasciitis.[2–5] Other diseases may be associated, including Achilles tendinitis, Charcot neuropathic arthropathy, recurrent ankle sprains, and many others.

The first step in identifying a contracted gastrocnemius-soleus complex is defining it. The best current definition is less than 10° of passive ankle dorsiflexion with the knee flexed and extended.[1,6,7] It is important to emphasize that the motion should be passive; passive motion accounts for the resting tone in the gastrocnemius, which must be considered. Active dorsiflexion using the anterior muscles turns off the resting tone in the gastrocnemius, giving improved dorsiflexion, but the important parameter to be measured is the dorsiflexion achievable in a simulated stance, where the anterior muscles are silent and gastrocnemius resting tone is relevant.

ANATOMY AND EVOLUTIONARY BASIS

Unlike the flexible primate foot used for grabbing tree branches, the human foot has a rigid longitudinal arch that links the forefoot to the hindfoot and transmits the energy

Department of Orthopedic Surgery, Columbia University Medical Center, 622 West 168th Street, PH11-Center, New York, NY 10032, USA
* Corresponding author.
E-mail address: JKG2101@columbia.edu (J. Greisberg).

Foot Ankle Clin N Am 14 (2009) 627–637
doi:10.1016/j.fcl.2009.08.002
1083-7515/09/$ – see front matter © 2009 Elsevier Inc. All rights reserved.

of a forceful Achilles tendon for propulsion.[8] When the heel cord or gastrocnemius contracture is present and an equinus deformity causes arch breakdown, foot dysfunction results.

Equinus contracture is a trait that has been referred to as atavistic by Hansen and others. The term atavistic suggests it is a reversion to a more primitive state, but it may be more appropriate to consider it incomplete evolution. Just about all vertebrates have a contracted Achilles tendon, so that the heel is held off the ground.[8,9] Because the gastrocnemius crosses the knee joint and the ankle, active extension of the knee during gait forces the ankle to plantarflex. Therefore, while running, a forceful knee extension will drive the ankle into plantarflexion and propel the animal efficiently.[10]

During the process of evolution from an arboreal primate ancestor to modern humans, the gastrocnemius-soleus has had to lengthen, to allow the heel to make contact with the ground. In the apes, the calcaneus remains relatively plantarflexed, but in the human, the calcaneus finally achieves a dorsiflexed position relative to the talus. The relative length of the gastrocnemius-soleus is polymorphic in the human population, with some humans having more tightness than may be ideal. A good example is often seen in sprinters and jumpers, who have marked tightness of the complex that serves them well during sport; they may gain quite a bit of propulsion.

Anatomically, the two heads of the gastrocnemius and the single soleus make up the triceps surae of the posterior compartment of the leg. The gastrocnemius muscle originates on the posterior aspect of the femoral condyles just proximal to the knee joint while the soleus muscle originates on the posterior superior aspect of the tibia. The Achilles tendon is the convergence of these muscles and inserts on the calcaneal tuberosity.[10,11] The gastrocnemius crosses the knee, ankle, and subtalar joints while the soleus crosses only the ankle and subtalar joint. This anatomy forms the basis for the Silfverskiold test.[12,13] Passive ankle dorsiflexion must be assessed with the knee both flexed and extended; if the ankle fails to reach 10° with the knee extended, but improves when the knee is flexed, it is the gastrocnemius only that is tight. If the ankle does not dorsiflex 10° in either knee position, then both muscles are contracted (**Fig. 1**) or an intrinsic ankle joint problem exists, such as capsular contracture, arthrosis, or fibrosis.

When examining the patient for Achilles contracture, it is essential to maintain a neutral reduction of the medial column or hindfoot. It is easy to shift the subtalar

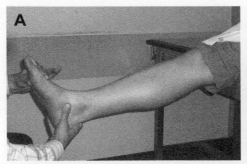
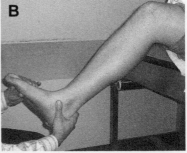

Fig. 1. (*A*) Equinus contracture is detected by first reducing the midfoot on the hindfoot by placing the examiner's thumb over the medial head of the talus while the opposite hand ensures neutral alignment of the forefoot and midfoot on the hindfoot. This ensures the relaxation of the anterior compartment muscles. Maximum dorsiflexion is noted. (*B*) The same is recorded with the knee flexed.

and talonavicular joints into valgus. Because of the oblique axis of those joints, valgus positioning will increase the perception of dorsiflexion, although the talus will still be plantarflexed. In other words, valgus positioning of the hindfoot will seem to increase dorsiflexion even in the presence of an Achilles contracture. This confounding variable is easily removed by simply maintaining the medial column (talonavicular joint) reduced in a neutral position (**Fig. 2**).

IMPLICATIONS OF TIGHT GASTROCNEMIUS

A functional equinus contracture is often due to gastrocnemius, not soleus, tightness. Gastrocnemius contractures can lead to muscle imbalance, gait disturbances, and progressive structural breakdown of the foot and ankle. Equinus deformities of the foot and ankle have been referred to as Achilles contractures; however, the majority of stretch in the posterior superficial compartment is due to the muscle bellies of the gastrocnemius and soleus and not the tendo-achilles complex. The tendon accounts for only 3% to 5% of the elastic stretch of the triceps surae.[1]

The calcaneal tuberosity, and thus the insertion of the Achilles, is normally in slight valgus and thus lateral to the long axis of the tibia. Contraction of the Achilles in this position pulls the subtalar and talonavicular joints into eversion. That is why it is so important for the posterior tibialis to fire before the Achilles in the heel-rise portion of gait. If the posterior tibialis does not fire, as in posterior tibial tendon dysfunction, the Achilles pulls the hindfoot into valgus and, over time, destroys the arch.[4]

A contracted gastrocnemius-soleus complex will encourage plantarflexion at the ankle when not weight bearing, but when the ground pushes up on the foot (in other words, when the foot strikes the ground), a contracted gastrocnemius will force the hindfoot into valgus, fatiguing the arch ligaments over time. Some have proposed that this is the first step in the adult-acquired flat foot, and the tibial tendon failure follows later.

A tight gastrocnemius may also be the culprit in plantar fasciitis and Achilles tendinitis. During the stance phase of gait, excess tightness in the gastrocnemius-soleus complex will increase tension in both the Achilles tendon and the plantar fascia. Some patients will sustain a pathologic degeneration of the Achilles tendon several centimeters above the insertion, and others will feel it at the insertion on the heel

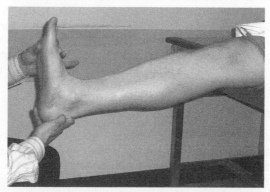

Fig. 2. Ensuring relaxation of the anterior muscles is essential in determining equinus contracture. If the midfoot is lateralized on the hindfoot, a falsely increased dorsiflexion is found by the firing of the anterior muscles and the reflex inhibition of the gastrocnemius-soleus complex.

(midsubstance versus insertional tendinosis). More commonly, the proximal plantar fascia will be affected.[2,11] For both Achilles tendinitis and plantar fasciitis, gastrocnemius stretching exercises have proven to be an effective treatment.[14]

Metatarsalgia can also be linked to a gastrocnemius contracture. The tight Achilles shifts plantar weight-bearing pressure from the hindfoot to the forefoot. In trying to overcome a strong triceps surae, the tibialis anterior may recruit the long toe extensors to help dorsiflex the ankle. Hyperextension at the metatarsalphalangeal joint occurs with resultant clawing of the toes. The shift in plantar pressure from the hindfoot to the forefoot, along with plantar fat pad migration (pulled distally by the claw toes) leads to forefoot pain. Patients with neuropathy may develop forefoot ulceration, and Achilles tendon lengthening has been shown to decrease the incidence of ulceration in these patients.[15]

Cadaveric studies have shown that the forefoot carries 20% of the weight-bearing load without loading the triceps surae. When 73 lbs of Achilles force is applied in the presence of 100 lbs of tibial weight bearing, forefoot weight bearing increased to 50%.[16] Another study confirmed this and found that plantar force increased in the forefoot and decreased in the hindfoot with increasing triceps surae force. The midfoot is similarly affected and Aronow and colleagues[11] noted a visual decrease in the medial longitudinal arch as triceps surae force is increased.

IMPLICATIONS OF A LOOSE GASTROCNEMIUS-SOLEUS COMPLEX

Too little tension in the musculotendinous complex will throw the muscle fibers off the peak of the length-tension curve (analogous to the Starling curve of cardiac muscle), with weakness as the result. The loose tendon may arise from an untreated Achilles rupture, or from denervation related to polio. It can also arise as a complication of surgical lengthening. Heel pain from a calcaneal deformity may be seen, owing to excessive weight transfer onto the heel. In diabetic patients with peripheral neuropathy and an insensate heel, plantar heel overload callus and ulcers can also develop, potentially leading to chronic calcaneal osteomyelitis.[17] Weakness in push off may cause a limp when walking, and exercise ability will be affected.[17] Although some low demand patients will not notice any trouble, the problems of the loose Achilles tendon are best avoided by prevention.

In severe cases, overlengthening of the calf results in a crouched or calcaneus gait.[15,18] The posterior triceps surae is too loose and weak to prevent the anterior translation of the tibia when the center of gravity moves anterior to the ankle during gait. This uncouples the normal ankle plantarflexion and knee extension and results in premature knee and hip flexion. The crouch gait increases the work of walking, decreases stride length, and patients experience early fatigue. Treatment of an over-lengthened triceps surae is difficult and the use of an anterior floor reaction brace in children with crouched gait has been described.[18]

TRICEPS SURAE LENGTHENING PROCEDURES

Conservative treatment options for equinus contracture includes physiotherapy with stretching exercises, night splints (subject to patient compliance), and serial casting (not currently used by most orthopedists). Functional orthosis can also be used for pressure redistribution and arch support. When nonoperative modalities fail, a number of operative triceps surae lengthening procedures exist, including open lengthening, percutaneous tendo-Achilles lengthening (PTAL), and proximal or distal gastrocnemius recessions. Numerous studies compare the different options with no clear consensus for the best procedure. The surgical choice depends upon each patient's individual pathology and surgeon preference. In planning a gastrocnemius-soleus lengthening, the Silverskjold test is the first step to determine if only the gastrocnemius, or the entire Achilles tendon, is tight.

Achilles Tendon Lengthening

In patients with Achilles tendon contractures, the tendon can be lengthened open or percutaneously. The essential concept is to lengthen adequately but not excessively. For open lengthening, a skin incision is made posteriorly, just medial to the Achilles tendon. The patient can be prone or supine. The tendon sheath is opened and preserved. A Z-lengthening is performed by first making a long longitudinal split down the center of the tendon. The tendon is divided by cutting either direction at the top and bottom of the slit, to complete the Z. The ankle is dorsiflexed to neutral with the knee extended and the foot is placed in neutral. The tendon is then sutured in tension using multiple horizontal mattress sutures. The paratenon, then the skin, are closed with meticulous technique to minimize adhesions. Once the skin has healed, the patient can be weight bearing in a cast or cast boot. By 8 weeks postoperatively, the patient may transition to a regular shoe, although sudden exertion on the tendon may need to be delayed for another month to minimize chance of rupture.

Percutaneous tendo-Achilles lengthening is another less invasive option for Achilles tendon lengthening. Hoke's technique of triple-cut hemisection is the standard by which most PTAL is performed.[19,20] The patient is placed supine. The foot is maximally dorsiflexed and elevated by the assistant to provide good visualization of the posterior leg and Achilles tendon. The tendon is palpated and the central one-third of the calcaneal tuberosity is identified at the insertion of the tendon. Three equidistant skin incisions are marked along the tendon. The minimum distance between incisions should be 3 cm. About 50% of the tendon is incised with each cut; the proximal and distal cuts are medial and the middle one is lateral, to minimize potential injury to the sural nerve. As these releases occur, an appreciable increase in ankle dorsiflexion is noted. A minimum of 90° of dorsiflexion and up to 10° to 15° past 90° with the knee extended is desirable. To prevent the possibility of complete rupture, correction of more than 30° should be avoided with this procedure.

An alternate technique of a two-incision PTAL is also effective. This technique takes advantage of the rotation of the collagen fibers in the tendon. Using the mnemonic DAMP, the distal incision is made just medial to the tendon and releases the anterior half. The proximal incision releases the medial half; then a noticeable lengthening is felt.[21]

An open lengthening has been proposed for more severe contractures, but the percutaneous technique is probably just as effective when there is no previous scarring. The open technique may create a risk for Achilles tendonosis because of significant scar tissue formation. An open lengthening requires more operative time and a larger scar as compared with percutaneous tendon lengthening. However, the amount of Achilles lengthening is more difficult to control with percutaneous method, and over lengthening is possible.

Iatrogenic Achilles rupture rate is also increased with PTAL and some advocate longer postoperative immobilization with protected weight bearing for 10 to 12 weeks followed by progressive weight bearing in a CAM (controlled ankle motion) walker for 2 to 4 weeks.

Gastrocnemius Recession

Numerous procedures have been described at differing anatomic levels for gastrocnemius recessions. In 1950, a more proximal recession was reviewed by Strayer.[22,23]

The Strayer recession separates the gastrocnemius from the soleus just proximal to the gastrocnemius-soleus aponeurosis and allows the transected gastrocnemius tendon to retract proximally. A 5 to 7 cm posteromedial skin incision is made along the lower leg just distal to the visible indentation of the gastrocnemius muscle and Achilles junction (**Fig. 3**). Dissection is carried through skin and subcutaneous fat down to the deep fascia, which is incised longitudinally. The saphenous nerve and vein may be in the subcutaneous tissue. An elevator is used to clear the subcutaneous fatty tissue off the gastrocnemius and the sural nerve identified if it is deep to the fascia. (In many patients, the nerve will have exited the fascia more proximally and may be superficial at this level.)

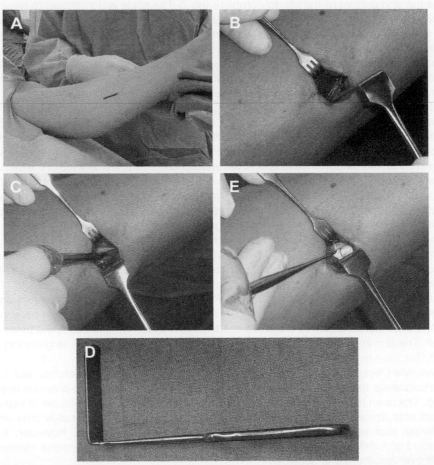

Fig. 3. (*A*) A longitudinal 3 cm posteromedial skin incision is made just distal to the gastrocnemius-soleus and Achilles junction. Dissection is carried through the subcutaneous fat down to the deep fascia, which is incised longitudinally. (*B*) The soleus muscle is first visualized anteriorly. (*C*) Blunt finger dissection separates the gastrocnemius-soleus interval medial to lateral. (*D*) A long right-angled Langenbeck rectractor is helpful to protect the posterior tissues (including the sural nerve). The gastrocnemius tendon is transected completely. (*E*) The plantaris tendon is palpated medially and released. The deep fascia is closed to prevent the tendon from adhering to the skin and puckering. The skin is closed last with a subcuticular stitch.

Blunt dissection separates the gastrocnemius-soleus interval medial to lateral. While protecting the posterior tissues (including the sural nerve) with a long right-angled retractor, the gastrocnemius tendon is transected completely. The surgeon must feel medially under the fascia to identify the plantaris tendon. If present, it should be released as well. The tendon edges will separate 1 to 2 cm; then the soleus will prevent any further retraction. It is helpful to close the deep fascia if there is no bleeding to prevent the tendon from adhering to the skin. The skin is closed with a careful technique to minimize scarring; we currently use a subcuticular stitch.

Even with careful technique, the scar may pucker or appear prominent in the calf. Sural neurapraxia is common, presumably because of stretch from retractors or, more likely, from increased stretch of the posterior muscles. Saphenous or sural nerve laceration is possible, but rare. In Pinney and colleagues report, approximately half of their patients had the sural nerve running superficial to the deep fascia, thereby protected during gastrocnemius recession.[7] In the other half, the sural nerve was found deep to the fascia and some specimens revealed a sural nerve that was adherent to the gastrocnemius tendon itself. The variability of sural nerve anatomy stresses the importance of correct identification and protection of the nerve before transaction of the gastrocnemius tendon.

The length of the posteromedial incision can also be minimized with correct identification of the junction of the gastrocnemius and Achilles tendon. Dissection is only needed proximally from this point. Pinney and colleagues[7] also showed that this junction was about 2 cm distal from the visible indent of the gastrocnemius. Therefore, the skin incision should start 2 cm distal to the visible indent. Some have used a pediatric speculum to isolate the gastrocnemius through a minimal incision.

Endoscopic Gastrocnemius Recession

Successful results have been reported with open gastrocnemius recessions; however, the desire for more cosmetically appealing scars has lead to the development of an endoscopic technique. Cadaveric studies have found complete gastrocnemius aponeurosis transection is possible with a two portal procedure and the mean improvement in ankle dorsiflexion is 20° with the knee in extension. However, visualization of the sural nerve can be difficult and lead to increased rates of iatrogenic nerve injury.[24]

Trevino and colleagues[25] reported their results on 31 endoscopic gastrocnemius recessions in 28 patients. Complications included two patients in whom the initial incision for the entry portal was at the wrong level, one in whom complete transaction of the gastrocnemius aponeurosis was not possible and had to be converted to an open procedure, and one with a superficial wound infection. There was no evidence of sural nerve injuries. Another study of 18 patients reported a 15% incidence of lateral foot dysesthesia.[26] Endoscopic technique may offer the promise of better cosmesis, but may come at the expense of slightly increased complications.

Proximal Gastrocnemius Recession

In addition to tendo-Achilles lengthening and gastrocnemius recession at the level of the gastrocnemius-soleus aponeurosis, more proximal procedures have also been described. The Silfverskiold operation is a gastrocnemius tenotomy at the level of the knee along with partial transection of the tibial motor nerves to the gastrocnemius muscle. Silver and Simon[13] later described the use of this procedure in children with cerebral palsy spastic equinus. Increased potential for neurovascular complications and the ability to gain the desired dorsiflexion with more distal and safer approaches have led most surgeons to lean away from such proximal releases. The Bauman procedure is a high gastrocnemius recession performed at the level of the medial and lateral heads. The patient is placed supine and the initial dissection is similar to a more distal recession. The interval between the gastrocnemius and soleus muscle is entered and a transverse incision is made through the entire gastrocnemius muscle fascia with transection of the intermuscular septum between the two heads. A parallel second recession, 1 to 2 cm distal, can also be done to further increase dorsiflexion. A major benefit of this proximal intramuscular lengthening is the preservation of muscle strength compared with more distal tendinous lengthening.[12]

SPECIFIC DISEASE STATES
Acquired Flatfoot

Achilles tightness is a deforming force that can exacerbate medial arch collapse. As the talus and calcaneus are plantarflexed, the subtalar joints evert to compensate and produce needed dorsiflexion. With subtalar eversion, the posterior tibialis tendon is strained, leading to further arch breakdown. A tight Achilles can also be a result of a low-arched feet; such a foot deformity may exacerbate a tight Achilles by maintaining the hindfoot in valgus. Once the deformity of a flatfoot occurs, it is difficult to distinguish the cause and effect relationship of an Achilles contracture or posterior tibial tendon dysfunction.[4] Surgical treatment for adult-acquired flatfoot should address all sources of pain and deformity including the tibial tendon failure, osseus deformity, and muscle imbalance. A gastrocnemius-soleus contracture falls under the category of muscle imbalance, and is universally present in the acquired flat foot. It may not be noticeable with the arch deformity, but once the hindfoot alignment is restored (by dorsiflexing the hindfoot relative to the midfoot), it is apparent.

An Achilles lengthening or gastrocnemius recession is indicated, depending on which is tight. Usually the stage 2 flat foot needs only a gastrocnemius recession, while the stage 3 flat foot often requires an entire Achilles tendon lengthening. We tend to perform the gastrocnemius recession at the beginning of a procedure, before tourniquet inflation. It is quite easy to do without a tourniquet. Percutaneous tendon lengthening is often done following realignment and screw fixation for the hindfoot fusion of the stage 3 flat foot.

Neuromuscular

Equinus deformity is the most common deformity in cerebral palsy and other spastic neuromuscular disorders. Physical therapy, bracing, and botulinum toxin injections are reasonable initial interventions. However, with marked Achilles contracture, surgery should be considered before arch collapse sets in, if possible. The type of lengthening procedure that is done is variable and frequently surgeon dependent. Given the complexity of the neuromuscular disorder and the effects of continued growth, equinus deformities frequently recur. In hemiplegia, the results are the most consistent and any of the methods of calf lengthening can be undertaken. Maintenance of the correction is rare and frequently necessitates relengthening. Diplegic and quadriplegic patients are more complex and may require concomitant hamstring and psoas lengthenings.[27]

However, there are some patients in which an equinus contracture is necessary. Patients with classic muscular dystrophy typically exhibit proximal limb weakness. Quadriceps weakness results in an inability to maintain the knee in extension while standing. To compensate, an equinus contracture develops. When the patient stands on a flat surface, the plantarflexed ankle will force the knee into hyperextension, thus locking the knee so that less quadriceps force is required to maintain knee extension.

In these patients, lengthening of the Achilles may result in the need for a knee-ankle-foot orthosis to stand.[28]

Diabetes

It has been noted that many patients with diabetes also have a gastrocnemius contracture. This increases plantar pressures under the metatarsal heads.[29] Forefoot ulceration is common in patients with diabetic neuropathy, and although total contact casting (TCC) has been shown to reduce pressure and is an effective treatment for ulceration, TCC is associated with a high rate of ulcer recurrence, from 20% to 70%.[30] Mueller and colleagues[5] in a randomized controlled trial compared the outcomes of patients with diabetic neuropathic ulcers who were treated with total contact casting alone and those with TCC and Achilles lengthening. They found that the recurrence rate of the group with TCC and Achilles tendon lengthening was 75% less than those who were treated only with TCC. Depending on the degree of tightness, gastrocnemius recession and percutaneous Achilles tendon lengthening are both effective methods for decreasing the risk of neuropathic ulcers. We tend to favor percutaneous Achilles lengthening in patients with forefoot ulceration.

In Charcot neuroarthropathy of the midfoot, the hindfoot plantarflexes relative to the midfoot. It seems likely that a contracted Achilles could be a contributing cause of the midfoot breakdown. Some advocate prophylactic gastrocnemius recession for any patient with diabetes.[31] Although not proven, given the tremendous expense and morbidity associated with diabetic foot disease, even if gastrocnemius recession is only marginally helpful it may be extremely cost effective for the diabetic at risk.

Plantar Fasciitis

The plantar fascia follows the insertion of the Achilles tendon on the heel and continues out to the plantar forefoot soft tissues. Tightness in the Achilles puts an increased strain on the plantar fascia with weight bearing; biomechanical studies have shown that an increase in Achilles tendon load results in reduction of the medial arch height and increased plantar fascia tension.[2] It is widely accepted that the tight Achilles is a culprit in the development of plantar fasciitis, and Achilles tendon stretching exercises are recommended universally.

Traditional surgical recommendations for recalcitrant plantar fasciitis include partial plantar fasciotomy.[14] However, if the pathology is primarily in the Achilles tendon, then perhaps an Achilles lengthening is more appropriate. Despite biomechanical studies linking a tight posterior compartment as an etiology of plantar fasciitis, there is currently no literature on the outcomes of gastrocnemius recession as a method of treatment for plantar fasciitis.

Our preferred technique is for gastrocnemius recession in patients with a tight gastrocnemius and a low arch, and partial plantar fasciotomy in those with less tightness in the gastrocnemius and a high or cavus arch.

Arthritis and Total Ankle Replacement

Achilles tendon contracture may be encountered during surgical treatment of ankle arthritis. Some cases of ankle arthritis are due to progressive valgus deformity of the acquired flatfoot. The first step in surgical treatment is to realign and fuse the hindfoot joints. Once the talus is dorsiflexed back into normal alignment, an equinus contracture will be evident. Usually a percutaneous Achilles lengthening is necessary at this step.[32]

When performing total ankle arthroplasty, the joint is opened with distraction to minimize bone resection. Once the implants are in place, the surgeon will often find the ankle will not dorsiflex to neutral; the increased height has created a relative contracture of the Achilles. Percutaneous lengthening can be helpful here also.

SUMMARY

Achilles contracture is a common finding and has been implicated in a number of pathologic conditions. The first step in dealing with the problem is in recognizing it. By studying comparative anatomy and evolutionary biology, it is easy to understand why gastrocnemius tightness is so prevalent. The physical examination must emphasize passive ankle dorsiflexion with the medial column reduced. Failure to achieve 10° of dorsiflexion with the knee flexed and extended suggests a contracture.

Treatment begins with stretching and other nonsurgical options, but surgical lengthening should be considered in any case where progress deformity is possible. Some surgeons have even recommended surgical lengthening in high-risk patients (diabetics) as soon as the contracture is identified, even before clinical problems.

REFERENCES

1. DiGiovanni CW, Kuo R, Tejwani N, et al. Isolated gastrocnemius tightness. J Bone Joint Surg Am 2002;84(6):962–70.
2. Cheung JT, Zhang M, An KN. Effect of Achilles tendon loading on plantar fascia tension in the standing foot. Clin Biomech (Bristol, Avon) 2006;21(2):194–203.
3. Deland JT. Adult-acquired flatfoot deformity. J Am Acad Orthop Surg 2008;16(7): 399–406.
4. Lobo M, Greisberg J. Adult acquired flatfoot. In: Di Giovanni C, Greisberg J, editors. Foot and ankle: core knowledge in orthopaedics, vol. 1. Philadelphia: Elsevier Mosby; 2007. p. 38–57.
5. Mueller MJ, Sinacore DR, Hastings MK, et al. Effect of Achilles tendon lengthening on neuropathic plantar ulcers. A randomized clinical trial. J Bone Joint Surg Am 2003;85(8):1436–45.
6. Pinney SJ, Hansen ST Jr, Sangeorzan BJ. The effect on ankle dorsiflexion of gastrocnemius recession. Foot Ankle Int 2002;23(1):26–9.
7. Pinney SJ, Sangeorzan BJ, Hansen ST Jr. Surgical anatomy of the gastrocnemius recession (Strayer procedure). Foot Ankle Int 2004;25(4):247–50.
8. Greisberg J. Foot and ankle anatomy and biomechanics. In: Di Giovanni C, Greisberg J, editors. Foot and ankle: core knowledge in orthopaedics, vol. 1. Philadelphia: Elsevier Mosby; 2007. p. 1–15.
9. Hansen ST Jr. Functional reconstruction of the foot and ankle. Baltimore (MD): Lippincott Williams & Wilkins; 2000.
10. Baddar A, Granata K, Damiano DL, et al. Ankle and knee coupling in patients with spastic diplegia: effects of gastrocnemius-soleus lengthening. J Bone Joint Surg Am 2002;84(5):736–44.
11. Aronow MS, Diaz-Doran V, Sullivan RJ, et al. The effect of triceps surae contracture force on plantar foot pressure distribution. Foot Ankle Int 2006;27(1):43–52.
12. Herzenberg JE, Lamm BM, Corwin C, et al. Isolated recession of the gastrocnemius muscle: the Baumann procedure. Foot Ankle Int 2007;28(11):1154–9.
13. Silver CM, Simon SD. Gastrocnemius-muscle recession (Silfverskiold operation) for spastic equinus deformity in cerebral palsy. J Bone Joint Surg Am 1959;41: 1021–8.
14. Neufeld SK, Cerrato R. Plantar fasciitis: evaluation and treatment. J Am Acad Orthop Surg 2008;16(6):338–46.

15. Chilvers M, Malicky ES, Anderson JG, et al. Heel overload associated with heel cord insufficiency. Foot Ankle Int 2007;28(6):687–9.
16. Jones R. The human foot: an experimental study of its mechanics, and the role of its muscles and ligaments in the support of the arch. Am J Anat 1941;68:1–38.
17. Delp SL, Statler K, Carroll NC. Preserving plantar flexion strength after surgical treatment for contracture of the triceps surae: a computer simulation study. J Orthop Res 1995;13(1):96–104.
18. Dietz FR, Albright JC, Dolan L. Medium-term follow-up of Achilles tendon lengthening in the treatment of ankle equinus in cerebral palsy. Iowa Orthop J 2006;26: 27–32.
19. Hoke M. An operation for the correction of extremely relaxed flat feet. J Bone Joint Surg Am 1939;13:773–83.
20. Lee WC, Ko HS. Achilles tendon lengthening by triple hemisection in adult. Foot Ankle Int 2005;26(12):1017–20.
21. Hoppenfeld S, deBoer P. Surgical exposures in orthopaedics: the anatomic approach. 3rd edition. Philadelphia: Lippincott Williams & Wilkins; 2003.
22. Strayer LM Jr. Recession of the gastrocnemius; an operation to relieve spastic contracture of the calf muscles. J Bone Joint Surg Am 1950;32(3):671–6.
23. Strayer LM Jr. Gastrocnemius recession; five-year report of cases. J Bone Joint Surg Am 1958;40(5):1019–30.
24. Tashjian RZ, Appel AJ, Banerjee R, et al. Endoscopic gastrocnemius recession: evaluation in a cadaver model. Foot Ankle Int 2003;24(8):607–13.
25. Trevino S, Gibbs M, Panchbhavi V. Evaluation of results of endoscopic gastrocnemius recession. Foot Ankle Int 2005;26(5):359–64.
26. Saxena A, Widtfeldt A. Endoscopic gastrocnemius recession: preliminary report on 18 cases. J Foot Ankle Surg 2004;43(5):302–6.
27. Borton DC, Walker K, Pirpiris M, et al. Isolated calf lengthening in cerebral palsy. Outcome analysis of risk factors. J Bone Joint Surg Br 2001;83(3):364–70.
28. Smith SE, Green NE, Cole RJ, et al. Prolongation of ambulation in children with Duchenne muscular dystrophy by subcutaneous lower limb tenotomy. J Pediatr Orthop 1993;13(3):336–40.
29. Maluf KS, Mueller MJ, Strube MJ, et al. Tendon Achilles lengthening for the treatment of neuropathic ulcers causes a temporary reduction in forefoot pressure associated with changes in plantar flexor power rather than ankle motion during gait. J Biomech 2004;37(6):897–906.
30. Myerson M, Papa J, Eaton K, et al. The total-contact cast for management of neuropathic plantar ulceration of the foot. J Bone Joint Surg Am 1992;74(2): 261–9.
31. Armstrong DG, Stacpoole-Shea S, Nguyen H, et al. Lengthening of the Achilles tendon in diabetic patients who are at high risk for ulceration of the foot. J Bone Joint Surg Am 1999;81(4):535–8.
32. Thomas RH, Daniels TR. Ankle arthritis. J Bone Joint Surg Am 2003;85(5):923–36.

Insertional Achilles Tendinosis: Pathogenesis and Treatment

Bryan D. Den Hartog, MD

KEYWORDS

- Achilles • Tendinosis • Flexor hallucis longus transfer
- Haglunds deformity • Insertional Achilles tendinosis

PATHOPHYSIOLOGY
Terminology

The terminology commonly used to describe Achilles tendon injury can be confusing and misleading. Although the term "tendonitis" is often used to depict tendon pain and swelling, inflammatory cells are infrequently seen in biopsy specimens of thickened and inflamed tendons except in association with tendon rupture. In reality, there seem to be various histopathologic entities that can cause Achilles tendon pain. The most common of these pathologies is tendinosis, which is a degenerative process without histologic or clinical signs of intratendinous inflammation. Many clinicians use the word "tendonitis" to describe a condition that is actually a tendinosis; this misnomer can lead to an underestimate of the chronicity of Achilles tendon injury. Paratenonitis is the state of acute edema and hyperemia of the paratenon, accompanied by the infiltration of inflammatory cells and the possible presence of fibrinous exudates filling the tendon sheath. A partial tear of the Achilles tendon refers to a visibly evident discontinuity of the tendon, which is not common acutely. Finally, Mafulli and colleagues[1-3] proposed that the combination of pain, swelling, and impaired performance be labeled "tendinopathy."

Incidence and Epidemiology

The occurrence of Achilles tendinopathy is highest among individuals who participate in middle- and long-distance running, track and field, tennis, badminton, volleyball, and soccer. Lysholm and Wiklander[4] reported an annual incidence of Achilles disorders between 7% and 9% in top-level runners. In studies with an extensive number of patients, the most common clinical diagnosis of Achilles disorders was tendinopathy (55%–66%) followed by insertional problems (retrocalcaneal bursitis

Black Hills Orthopedic and Spine Center, PO Box 6850, Rapid City, SD 57709–6850, USA
E-mail address: bryandenhartog@bhosc.com

Foot Ankle Clin N Am 14 (2009) 639–650
doi:10.1016/j.fcl.2009.08.005
1083-7515/09/$ – see front matter © 2009 Elsevier Inc. All rights reserved.

foot.theclinics.com

and insertional tendinopathy) (20%–25%). In a cohort study with 11 years of follow-up, Kujala and colleagues[5] reported that 79 (29%) of 269 male runners and 7 (4%) of 188 controls reported Achilles tendon overuse injury.

Kvist[6] studied the epidemiologic factors of Achilles tendon disorders in a large group of competitive and recreational athletes with Achilles tendon problems. In those reports, which consisted of 698 patients, 66% had Achilles tendinopathy and 23% had Achilles tendon insertional problems. The activities most associated with Achilles tendinopathy were distance running or running sports. Malalignment of the lower extremity was found in 60% of the patients with an Achilles tendon disorder.

Mechanism of Injury

Most Achilles tendon problems are related to a combination of mechanical pressure and possibly decreased vascularity and are multifactorial in origin.[7–9] The principal factors include host susceptibility and mechanical overload. The primary host factors are biomechanical malalignments and increasing age (with a presumed decrease in vascularity). Both hyperpronation and cavus foot have been associated with Achilles tendon problems. Marked forefoot varus has been found to be more common in athletes with Achilles paratenonitis and insertional complaints. The cavus foot has also been associated with a high rate of insertional difficulties. The cavus foot is thought to absorb shock poorly and to place more stress on the lateral side of the Achilles tendon.

Advancing age has been shown to correlate with Achilles tendon overuse injuries. It has been hypothesized that decreased tendon vascularity associated with aging is the basis for the association of tendinopathy with age. Recent studies using laser Doppler flowmetry, however, have brought this commonly espoused theory into question.[10,11] Several mechanical factors have been implicated as part of the multifactorial etiology of Achilles tendon problems. Inappropriate footwear with insufficient heel height, rigid soles, inadequate shock absorption, or wedging from uneven wear can magnify the stresses exerted on the tendon during activity. Training errors include sudden increases in training intensity; excessive training; training on hard surfaces; and running on sloping, hard, or slippery roads. A change in training schedule shortly before injury has been recorded in as many as 50% of running injuries.[12]

CLASSIFICATION

Various classification schemes exist (**Box 1**).[13] Tendinopathies more than likely represent a continuum, however, with retrocalcaneal bursitis being the mild form and advanced calcific tendinosis the most severe form.

DIAGNOSIS
Patient History

The patient's history should provide most of the information to make the diagnosis of Achilles tendinopathy. The time interval between the onset of symptoms and the first visit to a physician, and the onset of the symptoms, the injury mechanism in patients with an acute case, and possible previous Achilles tendon problems and their treatment must be recorded. The course of events since the onset of symptoms, with special emphasis on the activities that seem to make the pain worse and the interventions that seem to relieve the pain, provide valuable additional information.

Pain is the cardinal symptom of Achilles tendinopathy that leads a patient to seek medical help, and it is the most common measure used to classify the severity of the disorder. It has been suggested that the patient's symptoms can reflect the degree

Box 1
Classification scheme of Puddu and coworkers
Paratenonitis
Tendinosis
Partial rupture
Paratenonitis with tendinosis
Degeneration
Partial tears
Calcification
Insertional tendinitis
Retrocalcaneal bursitis
Haglund deformity
Tendo Achilles bursitis
Complete rupture
Acute
Chronic
Data from Puddu G, Ippolito E, Postacchini F. A classification of Achilles tendon disease. Am J Sports Med 1976;4:145–50; with permission.

of the tendon abnormality. Patients in the early phase primarily report that they have pain following strenuous activities, whereas those in the later phase report that pain accompanies all activities and may even occur at rest. At this stage, the patient is usually unable to perform sports.

Physical Examination

The physical examination should follow the classic orthopedic scheme of "look, feel, and move." Inspection and palpation should provide a record of the contour of the muscle-tendon unit, possible areas of swelling and crepitation, increased erythema, local heat, and palpable tendon nodules or defects. In addition, patients with symptoms of Achilles tendinopathy should be examined for ankle instability and biomechanical faults.

In the acute phase of the Achilles tendinopathy, the tendon is diffusely swollen and, on palpation, tenderness is usually greatest in its distal third. Sometimes, crepitation can be palpated.

In the more chronic phase of Achilles tendinopathy, exercise-induced pain is still the cardinal symptom, whereas crepitation and swelling diminish. In patients with a chronic case a tender, nodular swelling is usually present and is believed to signify tendinosis. Particularly in patients with tendinosis, the focal tender nodules may move as the ankle is dorsiflexed and plantar flexed.

Imaging

The two modalities that can best image the Achilles tendon are sonography and MRI. Recent refinements in both technologies have tremendously improved the ability to image pathologic changes in tendons. Each technique has its inherent advantages and disadvantages.

Sonography is relatively inexpensive, is fast and repeatable, and has the potential for dynamic examination. It does, however, require substantial experience to learn how to operate the probe and interpret the images correctly. It is most reliable in determining the thickness of the Achilles tendon and the size of a gap after a complete rupture.

In contrast to sonography, MRI is relatively expensive and is typically not used for dynamic assessment. It is superior in the detection of incomplete tendon ruptures and the evaluation of various stages of chronic degenerative changes. It can also be used to monitor tendon healing when recurrent partial rupture is suspected.

TREATMENT OPTIONS

Treatment should be initially directed toward relieving symptoms. This should consist of a combination of nonoperative strategies aimed at controlling inflammation and correcting training errors, limb malalignment, decreased flexibility, muscle weakness, and avoiding the use of poor equipment during sports.[8]

Control of inflammation is recommended in the early phase of Achilles tendon overuse injury by decreasing activity, the use of cold packs, and the administration of anti-inflammatory medication. Shoe modifications include soft heels or heel elevation to pull the insertion away from the posterior tuberosity or an open heeled shoe, such as a clog, to reduce direct pressure on the Achilles insertion.

Rest, cross-training by decreasing the intensity, frequency, and duration of the activity that caused the injury, or modification of that activity, may be the only action needed to control the inflammation and symptoms in the acute phase. Modified rest, which allows activity in the uninjured parts of the body, such as the upper extremities, has been recommended. Casting for 3 to 4 weeks can be helpful in some patients who are acutely inflamed.

Cryotherapy has been regarded as the single most useful intervention for tendon inflammation in the acute phase of this disorder. Nonsteroidal anti-inflammatory drugs, in the form of pills or topical gels, are frequently used in the treatment of acute and chronic forms of Achilles tendinopathy. The benefit of these drugs is, however, controversial. Although healing of acute soft tissue injury is slightly more rapid and inflammation is slightly better controlled with the use of nonsteroidal anti-inflammatory drugs, they seem to have no benefit in the advanced stages of tendinosis.

Corticosteroid injections in the treatment of Achilles tendinopathy are controversial because there are insufficient published data to determine the comparative benefits and risks. In general, caution should be used when using corticosteroids around the Achilles insertion because of the theoretical concern of acute Achilles rupture.

Eccentric stretching and strengthening of the triceps surae muscle and the Achilles tendon have been advocated to preserve the function of the musculo-tendinous unit by restoring normal ankle joint mobility and decreasing the strain of the Achilles tendon with normal motion.[14] Alfredson[11] demonstrated the benefit of eccentric calf-muscle training in patients with chronic insertional Achilles tendon pain.

Physical therapy modalities, such as heat, ultrasound, electrical stimulation, and laser photo stimulation, are commonly used in the treatment of Achilles tendinopathy. Scientific evidence on the effectiveness of these treatment modalities is sparse and controversial, especially with regard to the long-term clinical benefits.

SURGICAL TREATMENT

Surgical intervention is considered for chronic cases of insertional Achilles tendinosis (IAT) if the treatment is resistant to an exhaustive nonoperative program. Various surgical techniques have been used to treat Achilles tendinopathy. Most involve removal of inflamed or diseased tissue and decompression of mechanical pressure from the adjacent calcaneus.

Contraindications for surgical treatment include patients with skin or vascular compromise or those with minimal pain. Some studies have shown a relatively high rate of complications associated with operative treatment of Achilles tendinopathy.[6] Recently, an overall complication rate of 11% was documented in a series of 432 consecutive patients.[15,16] Most of the complications (54%) in that study involved compromised wound healing, and the problem seemed to appear more frequently in patients who had operative treatment of a partial Achilles tendon rupture than in those who only had operative treatment of Achilles tendinopathy.

Overview of Treatment Options

Excision of degenerative tendon

When an intratendinous lesion is seen on preoperative ultrasonography or MRI examination and a nodule or thickening is palpable within the tendon, many authors have recommended that a longitudinal incision be made over the thickened area and the necrotic area or granulation tissue be excised. If a large segmental gap remains after tendon debridement, a turned-down tendon flap has been proposed to reinforce the tendon if there is a need to bridge the gap after extensive debridement.[17] Alternatively, some authors have used multiple longitudinal incisions of the tendon to treat this condition.[2]

Decompression of impinging bone

Removal of the posterosuperior aspect of the calcaneus (the Haglund deformity) to decompress the Achilles insertion can be done alone for early stages of tendinopathy or more commonly in combination with excision of the degenerated portion of the Achilles insertion.[18,19]

Augmentation of the debrided Achilles with the flexor hallucis longus tendon

The flexor hallucis longus (FHL) tendon is used to bring mechanical support to the remaining Achilles' segment after thorough tendon debridement.[20–25] Although other tendons are available for transfer,[26] advantages of the FHL (flexor digitorum longus, peroneus brevis) include stronger plantarflexion, an axis of contracture more in line with the Achilles, an in-phase firing with the gastrocsoleus complex, and its anatomic proximity to the Achilles.

Complete detachment of the Achilles from the calcaneus with reattachment and augmentation

In some patients, it may be necessary to debride most or all of the Achilles' insertion. If less than 2 cm of tendon length is removed during the debridement, the remaining insertion can be reattached with suture anchors after the FHL has been transferred. If the gap is greater than 2 cm, tendon augmentation, such as a gastrocnemius turndown flap with FHL transfer, or FHL transfer alone, may be necessary to bridge the tendon gap.[27–30]

TECHNIQUE

The FHL transfer is indicated for those patients with chronic, disabling pain who have failed 6 or more months of nonoperative treatment. Contraindications include patients with skin compromise and reduced vascularity.

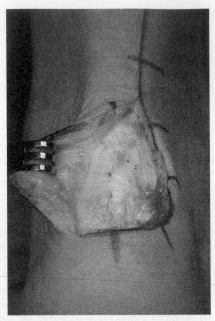

Fig. 1. The posteromedial incision with and transverse extension that improves exposure of the diseased tendon.

There are some pearls to remember. Full-thickness incision to paratenon should be made without undermining skin. This reduces risk of skin necrosis. All diseased tissue should be excised. Leaving behind degenerative tendon increases risk of persistent pain postoperatively.

If FHL transfer is indicated, harvest the tendon from behind the ankle through the same incision and avoid making a separate incision at the midfoot. In most patients, one does not need the extra tendon length and the extra incision adds time, risk, and increased morbidity to the procedure. Anchoring the FHL transfer can be done with 5-mm suture anchors or with an interference screw through a bone tunnel if enough length of the transferred tendon is available.

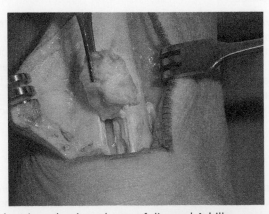

Fig. 2. Excision of the triangular-shaped area of diseased Achilles.

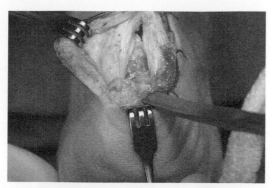

Fig. 3. Remove the posterior spur at the insertion of the Achilles.

Pitfalls to watch for include leaving unhealthy tissue behind, and having persistent pain and wound healing problems if skin edges are undermined.

OPERATIVE PROCEDURE

Place the patient prone on the operating table under general or spinal anesthesia. A posterior medial incision is made along the diseased Achilles and brought down sharply through the paratenon (**Fig. 1**). The horizontal extension of the distal portion of the posteromedial incision is done at the distal Achilles insertion to give better exposure of the diseased tissue. Care must be taken to not undermine the skin edges.

The diseased segment of tendon is incised (usually in a triangular fashion) and the degenerative portions are identified and excised (**Fig. 2**). One should go to where the lesion is, usually at the central insertion. The abnormal tendon has a "codfish flesh," which is identified by its homogenous appearance and loss of the normal collagen striations. The calcific spur at the insertion of the Achilles is removed with an osteotome (**Fig. 3**).

If most of the cross-sectional area of the tendon remains, closure of the tendon or paratenon is done. If greater than 50% of the cross-sectional area is resected, consider augmenting the repair. Up to 50% of insertion of Achilles can probably be removed before risking rupture postoperatively.[31]

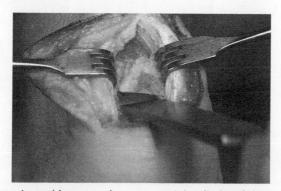

Fig. 4. An osteotome is used between the two remaining limbs of the Achilles insertion to remove the Haglund deformity.

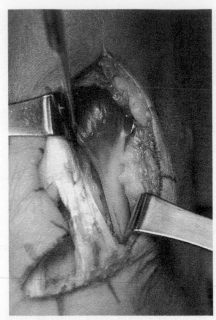

Fig. 5. The FHL is exposed through an extension of the incision proximally.

To make room for the transfer, the posterosuperior tuberosity of the calcaneus is removed with an osteotome (**Fig. 4**). One should make sure enough bone is removed to prevent further impingement on Achilles with the ankle dorsiflexed.

If augmentation of the debrided Achilles is warranted, the FHL is the preferred transfer because of its strength and proximity. The FHL is harvested through the posteromedial incision by excising the fat pad in front of the Achilles and splitting the deep fascia to expose the FHL, which lies directly behind the ankle and subtalar joints.

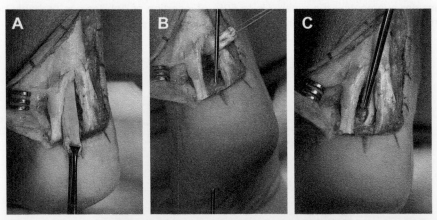

Fig. 6. (*A*) The transected FHL tendon is pulled distally to assess for adequate length for bone tunnel fixation. (*B*) A guidewire for the bone tunnel is placed between the limbs of the remaining Achilles. (*C*) The interference screw is placed with the FHL under proper tension.

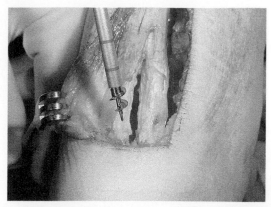

Fig. 7. A 5-mm double-strand cork screw anchor is placed in the hard cancellous bone near the normal insertion of the Achilles.

Once the FHL is identified, it is dissected as far distal as possible while plantar flexing the ankle and great toe. A retractor is placed medial to the tendon to protect the neurovascular bundle (**Fig. 5**). The FHL is then cut medial to lateral, cutting away from the posterior tibial nerve.

The ankle is then maximally dorsiflexed and the FHL is brought alongside the Achilles. The appropriate length of the FHL is determined, and if the tendon length is sufficient, the tendon can be secured by using an interference screw through a bone tunnel (**Fig. 6**). If the transferred tendon is too short for a bone tunnel fixation, it is anchored to the calcaneus with a double-stranded 5-mm corkscrew anchor (**Fig. 7**). If a double-stranded 5-mm corkscrew anchor is used, the first suture is placed at the end of the transferred tendon to secure the FHL in a position just anterior to the Achilles in the exposed cancellous bone of the calcaneus. The second suture strand is placed up each side of the FHL in a whip-stitch fashion to add pullout strength (**Fig. 8**).

The FHL is sutured side-to-side to the Achilles with a nonabsorbable braided suture (**Fig. 9**). Dorsiflexion is then checked to make sure that the preoperative range of motion (ROM) has not been compromised. Marcaine 0.5% is injected in and around the surgical site. Either a well-padded cast or Jones dressing is placed with the ankle in neutral.

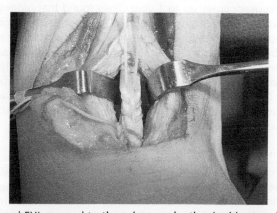

Fig. 8. The transferred FHL secured to the calcaneus by the double-stranded suture anchor.

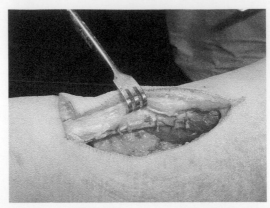

Fig. 9. The transferred FHL is sutured side-to-side to the remaining Achilles.

POSTOPERATIVE CARE

A short leg cast or bulky Jones' dressing is applied in the operating room and the patient kept at toe-touch weight bearing for 2 to 4 weeks or until the incision is well healed. A controlled ankle motion (CAM) soled walker is applied and weight-bearing as tolerated is allowed. The patient can begin weaning the boot as the pain and swelling decrease (usually 4–6 weeks).

RESULTS

In most studies, operative treatment of Achilles tendinopathy has given satisfactory results in 75% to 100% of the patients. Many of these reports are retrospective, however, and only a few had results that were based on objective evaluations, such as range of motion of the ankle. Next is a summary of reported results from the various types of treatment for IAT.

Debridement Alone

Several authors have reported satisfactory or good results from removal of diseased tissue and decompression with resection of the Haglund deformity.[16,19,31,32] Most had good pain relief with return to weight bearing and activity in 2 to 3 months, but some still had lengthy recovery times up to 1 year. They found that older patients still had difficulty with residual pain, problems with shoe wear, and return to prior activity level. Some patients had prolonged recovery times of 1 to 2 years. Watson and colleagues[31] reported a 93% patient satisfaction with debridement for retrocalcaneal bursitis and 74% with debridement alone for IAT, but noted that patients with IAT and calcification were older, had longer recovery, more pain, and shoe wear restrictions. They noted that patients over 55 years of age did not have as good an outcome with debridement alone. The IAT patient group had a 41% complication rate. In general, these studies tend to suggest using this treatment in younger patients.

Debridement with FHL Augmentation

Several authors have reported good or excellent relief on pain in those patients with advanced IAT, even in those patients over 50 years of age who seem to have poorer results with debridement alone.[20,23,24,30] Wapner and coworkers[21] were the first to study the results of the FHL transfer and found six of seven patients had good relief of their pain. Den Hartog[23] reported good or excellent results in 26 of 29 patients with tendinosis refractory to nonoperative treatment. Martin and colleagues[29] reported good or excellent pain relief and no loss of plantarflexion strength or power in 40 patients with an average follow-up of 27 months. They concluded that operative repair using an FHL autograft with a single incision technique achieved a high percentage of satisfactory results and excellent functional and clinical outcomes including significant pain relief.

The sacrifice of the FHL through the single incision with loss of plantarflexion of the great toe interphalangeal joint does not seem to cause any significant postoperative morbidity.[33]

SUMMARY

Insertional Achilles tendinopathy can be a painful debilitating condition that should initially be treated nonoperatively. If pain becomes chronic and debilitating, despite appropriate conservative treatment, debridement of the diseased portion of the Achilles tendon and removal of the impinging calcaneal prominence and transfer of the FHL through a single incision can be a reliable pain-relieving procedure with relatively high patient satisfaction.

REFERENCES

1. Maffulli N, Khan KM, Pudda G. Overuse tendon conditions: time to change a confusing terminology. Arthroscopy 1998;14:840–3.
2. Maffulli N. Current concepts review: rupture of the Achilles tendon. J Bone Joint Surg Am 1999;81:1019–36.
3. Maffulli N, Kader D. Tendinopathy of tendon Achilles. J Bone Joint Surg Br 2002; 84:1–8.
4. Lysholm J, Wiklander J. Injuries in runners. Am J Sports Med 1987;15:168–71.
5. Kujala UM, Sarna S, Kaprio J. Cumulative incidence of Achilles tendon rupture and tendinopathy in male former elite athletes. Clin J Sport Med 2005;15:133–5.
6. Kvist M. Achilles tendon injuries in athletes. Am J Sports Med 1994;18:173–201.
7. Saltzman C, Tearse D. Achilles tendon injuries. J Am Acad Orthop Surg 1998;6: 316–25.
8. Sorosky B, Press J, Plastaras C, et al. The practical management of Achilles tendinopathy. Clin J Sport Med 2004;14:40–4.
9. Paavola M, Kannus P, Jarvinen TA, et al. Achilles tendinopathy. J Bone Joint Surg Am 2002;84:2062–76.
10. Alfredson H, Ohberg L, Forsgren S. Is vasculo-neural ingrowth the cause of pain in chronic Achilles tendinosis? Knee Surg Sports Traumatol Arthrosc 2003;11:334–8.
11. Alfredson H. Chronic midportion Achilles tendinopathy: an update on research and treatment. Clin Sports Med 2003;22:727–41.
12. Schepsis A, Jones H, Haas A. Achilles tendon disorders in athletes. Am J Sports Med 2002;30:287–305.
13. Pudda G, Ippolito E, Postacchini F. A classification of Achilles tendon disease. Am J Sports Med 1976;4:145.
14. Fahlstrom M, Jonsson P, Lorentzon R, et al. Chronic Achilles tendon pain treated with eccentric calf-muscle training. Knee Surg Sports Traumatol Arthrosc 2003; 11:327–33.
15. Schepsis AA,, Leach RE. Surgical management of Achilles tendonitis. Am J Sports Med 1987;15(4):308–15.

16. Schepsis AA, Wagner C, Leach RE. Surgical management of Achilles tendon overuse injuries: a long term follow up study. Am J Sports Med 1994;22:611–9.
17. Den Hartog BD. Surgical strategies: delayed diagnosis or neglected Achilles tendon ruptures. Foot Ankle Int 2008;29:456–63.
18. Johnson KW, Zalavaras C, Thordardson DB. Surgical management of insertional calcific Achilles tendinosis with a central tendon splitting incision approach. Foot Ankle Int 2006;27(4):245–50.
19. McGarvey WC, Palumbo RC, Baxter DE, et al. Insertional Achilles tendinosis: surgical treatment through a central tendon splitting approach. Foot Ankle Int 2002;23:19–25.
20. Hanson ST. Trauma to the heel cord. In: Jahss MH, editor. Disorders of the foot and ankle. 2nd edition. Philadelphia: W.B. Saunders; 1991. p. 2357.
21. Wapner KL, Pavlock GS, Hecht PJ, et al. Repair of chronic Achilles tendon rupture with flexor hallucis longus tendon transfer. Foot Ankle 1993;14:443–9.
22. Den Hartog BD. Use of proximal flexor hallucis longus transfer in severe calcific Achilles' tendinosis. Tech Foot Ankle Surg 2002;1(2):145–50.
23. Den Hartog BD. Flexor hallucis longus tendon transfer for chronic Achilles tendinosis. Foot Ankle Int 2003;24(3):233–7.
24. Wilcox DK, Bohay DR, Anderson JG. Treatment of chronic Achilles tendon disorders with flexor hallucis longus transfer/augmentation. Foot Ankle Int 2000;21(12):1004–10.
25. Hahn F, Meyer P, Maiwald C, et al. Treatment of chronic Achilles tendinopathy and ruptures with flexor hallucis tendon transfer: clinical outcome and MRI findings. Foot Ankle Int 2008;29:794–802.
26. Turco VJ, Spinella AJ. Achilles tendon rupture-peroneus brevis transfer. Foot Ankle 1987;7:253–9.
27. Wagner E, Gould JS, Bilen E, et al. Change in plantar flexion strength after complete detachment and reconstruction of the Achilles tendon. Foot Ankle Int 2004;25(11):800–4.
28. Wagner E, Gould JS, Kneidal M, et al. Technique and results of Achilles tendon detachment and reconstruction for insertional Achilles tendinosis. Foot Ankle Int 2006;27(9):677–84.
29. Martin RL, Manning CM, Carcia CR, et al. An outcome study of chronic Achilles tendinosis after excision of the Achilles tendon and flexor hallucis longus tendon transfer. Foot Ankle Int 2005;26(9):691–7.
30. Elias I, Besser M, Nazarian LN, et al. Reconstruction for missed or neglected Achilles tendon rupture with V-Y lengthening and flexor hallucis transfer through one incision. Foot Ankle Int. 2007;28(12):1238–48.
31. Watson AD, Anderson RB, Davis HW. Comparison of results of retrocalcaneal decompression for retrocalcaneal bursitis and insertional Achilles tendinosis with calcific spur. Foot Ankle Int 2000;21:638–42.
32. Tallon C, Coleman BD, Khan KM, et al. Outcome of surgery for chronic Achilles tendinopathy. Am J Sports Med 2001;29:315–20.
33. Coull R, Flavin R, Stephens MM. Flexor hallucis longus tendon transfer: evaluation of postoperative morbidity. Foot Ankle Int 2003;12:931–4.

Surgical Treatment of Non-Insertional Achilles Tendinitis

G. Andrew Murphy, MD

KEYWORDS

• Achilles tendon • Tendinitis • Non-insertional • Surgery

Many different pathologic conditions can exist and even coexist in the Achilles tendon, and the terminology often is confusing. In addition to tendinitis, other terms used to describe pathologic conditions in the Achilles tendon include tenosynovitis, tendinosis, peritendinitis, tendinopathy, and peritendinopathy. These conditions are differentiated by cause, inflammation or degeneration; by structure affected, in the tendon body or localized to the peritenon; by location in the tendon, insertional or non-insertional; and by chronicity, acute or chronic. Some have suggested that "tendinitis" is an inappropriate term for the Achilles tendon, because its relative avascularity makes it resistant to an inflammatory response and histologic studies have shown either absent or minimal inflammation.[1-4] Rees and colleagues[4-6] suggested that inflammation may play a role in the initiation of the disease process but not in its propagation and progression. "Tendinopathy" has been suggested as a more appropriate term to describe the clinical conditions of pain and pathologic changes that occur in and around the tendon.[4-6]

Classifications of Achilles tendon pathology have been based on the duration of symptoms[7]: acute, symptoms for less than 2 weeks; subacute, symptoms for 3 to 6 weeks; and chronic, symptoms for longer than 6 weeks. Another classification[8] divided Achilles tendon dysfunction into insertional tendinitis (within or around the tendon at its calcaneal insertion) and non-insertional tendinitis (proximal to the tendon insertion within or on the tendon periphery). Puddu and colleagues[9] described 3 stages of tendon pathology: peritendinitis (stage 1), with pathologic changes localized to the peritenon; peritendinitis with tendinosis (stage 2), with involvement of peritendinous structures and tendon degeneration; and tendinosis (stage 3), with asymptomatic degeneration of the tendon without concomitant inflammation (**Tables 1 and 2**).

Department of Orthopaedic Surgery, Campbell Clinic, University of Tennessee, Memphis, Tennessee, 1211 Union Avenue, Suite 510, Memphis, TN 38104, USA
E-mail address: gmurp@earthlink.net

Foot Ankle Clin N Am 14 (2009) 651–661
doi:10.1016/j.fcl.2009.08.008
1083-7515/09/$ – see front matter © 2009 Elsevier Inc. All rights reserved.

foot.theclinics.com

Table 1
Classification of Achilles tendinopathy
Peritendinitis: inflammation involving peritendinous structures
Thickening of peritenon
Fluid accumulation adjacent to tendon
Development of adhesions
Peritendinitis with tendinosis: inflammation of peritendinous structures + degenerative changes
Macroscopic tendon thickening, nodularity
Softening
Yellowing
Fibrillation
Focal degeneration within tendon
Tendinosis: asymptomatic degeneration without inflammation caused by accumulated microtrauma, aging, or both
Degenerative lesions without evidence of peritendinitis
Altered tendon structure
Decreased luster
Yellowish discoloration
Softening

From Puddu G, Ippolito E, Postachini F. A classification of Achilles tendon disease. Am J Sports Med 1976;4:145–50; with permission.

PATHOPHYSIOLOGY

Several possible causes have been suggested for Achilles tendinopathy, including overuse (although tendinopathy also occurs in inactive individuals), decreased blood supply and tensile strength with aging, muscle imbalance or weakness, insufficient flexibility, and malalignment (hyperpronation); however, most of these theories are based on poor scientific evidence. Biopsies of affected Achilles tendons have revealed cellular activation and increases in cell numbers and ground substance, collagen disarray, and neovascularization.[10–12] Although prostaglandin inflammatory elements are not present, neurogenic inflammatory elements, such as substance P and calcitonin gene-related peptide, have been isolated.[13,14] Neovascular ingrowth and glutamate (a potent modulator of pain) have been noted in diseased tendons and have been postulated to be the source of pain in patients with Achilles tendinopathy.[13–15] With normal aging, the Achilles tendon undergoes substantial morphologic changes, including decreased cell density, decreased collagen fibril diameter and density, and loss of fiber waviness, all of which may contribute to more frequent Achilles tendon disorders in older athletes.[16,17] Some recent data support a genetic factor in the development of Achilles tendinopathy.[18]

ANATOMIC CONSIDERATIONS

The Achilles tendon is the longest and strongest tendon in the human body, inserting over a broad area (approximately 2 × 2 cm) on the posterosuperior aspect of the calcaneal tuberosity.[19] The gastrocnemius-soleus (triceps surae) muscle complex crosses the ankle and knee joints; the gastrocnemius serves as an ankle plantar flexor when the knee is extended, with the soleus, which crosses only the ankle joint, being

Table 2
Peritendinitis versus peritendinitis with tendinosis versus tendinosis with acute complete rupture

	Peritendinitis	Peritendinitis with Tendinosis (Partial Rupture)	Tendinosis with Acute Complete Rupture
Pain	Acute	Subacute/chronic	Acute
Audible snap or pop	None	Unlikely	+
Muscle weakness	+	+	+
Antalgic gait	+	+	+
Edema	+	+	+
Pain with palpation	+	+	+
Tendon gap	-	±	+
Tendon crepitus	±	±	-
Passive dorsiflexion excursion	Decreased	Decreased	Increased
Thompson test	-	-	+
Calf atrophy	-	+	±
Single-limb toe-rise	+	±	Unable to perform
Plantarflexion strength	Decreased	Decreased	Severely decreased

Modified from Coughlin MJ, Schon LC. Disorders of tendons. In: Coughlin MJ, Mann RA, Saltzman CL, editors. Surgery of the Foot and Ankle, 8th edition. Philadelphia: Mosby/Elsevier; 2007. p. 1224; with permission.

a more effective plantar flexor when the knee is flexed. The Achilles tendon has no true synovial sheath, but below the musculotendinous junction, the tendon is encased in a peritenon of varying thickness. The vascular supply to the tendon comes from the calcaneus distally through interosseous arterioles, proximally from intramuscular arterial branches, and on the anterior (deep) side of the tendon, from the mesotenon.[20,21] A zone of relative avascularity has been identified 2 to 6 cm proximal to the calcaneal insertion,[20,22] a characteristic that seems to predispose the Achilles tendon to degenerative changes in this area.

EXAMINATION

A careful history is important in the evaluation of the patient with Achilles tendinitis. Questions should be asked about an injury or a series of small injuries, a change in activity level or initiation of new sports. Activities such as walking on an inclined treadmill, a hilly area, or on the curved shoulder of the road may provide a clue to mechanical reasons for the problem. Any new medical problems or medications, specifically fluoroquinolones, should be queried. The physical examination should be made with the patient sitting, standing, and prone, and with the patient walking to provide a visual gait analysis. The following should also be assessed: (1) When sitting, does the patient have a selective gastrocnemius contracture or atrophy? (2) Is there restriction of subtalar motion? (3) Does the patient have normal strength? (4) Is there any cutaneous evidence of systemic disease? (5) Is knee motion and alignment normal? (6) When standing, what is the hindfoot position? (7) Are leg lengths equal? (8) Are the calves symmetric? (9) When lying prone, is the tenderness localized? (10) With ankle dorsiflexion and plantarflexion, does the pain move with the tendon (tendinosis), or does it stay in the same position (peritendinitis with or without tendinosis; **Fig. 1**)? (11) Is the equinus posture of the involved ankle equal to the other ankle? (12) Is the Thompson test result positive?

Plain radiographic examination usually is unproductive, but occasionally soft-tissue swelling or calcifications in the tendon are seen. Ultrasound examination may show fluid around the tendon or hypoechoic areas of tendon degeneration. Magnetic resonance imaging (MRI) is the test of choice at the author's institution because of its ability to quantify the amount of intratendinous degeneration or tenosynovitis (**Fig. 2**).

NONSURGICAL TREATMENT

Nonsurgical treatment is almost always the initial treatment of Achilles tendinitis, with surgical treatment recommended if there is no response within 3 to 6 months.[23] One

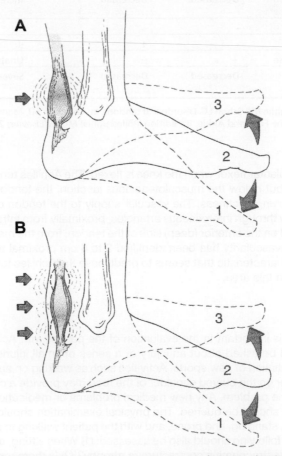

Fig. 1. With peritendinitis (*A*), tenderness remains in one location despite dorsiflexion and plantar flexion of the ankle. With tendinosis (*B*), this is the point of maximal tenderness proximally and distally as the ankle is dorsiflexed and plantar flexed. (*From* Coughlin MJ, Schon LC. Disorders of tendons. In: Coughlin MJ, Mann RA, Saltzman CL, editors. Surgery of the Foot and Ankle, 8th edition. Philadelphia: Mosby/ Elsevier; 2007. p. 1224; with permission.)

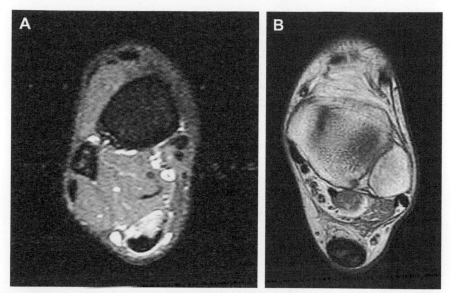

Fig. 2. (A) Peritendinous fluid characterizes tendinitis with minimal tendinosis in this T2-weighted MRI. (B) Extensive tendinosis is evident in this MRI of a 44-year-old runner.

8-year study of 83 patients with acute to subacute Achilles tendinopathy found that nonsurgical treatment was unsuccessful in almost one-third[24]; another found that 51% of patients improved with an average of 18 weeks of nonsurgical therapy.[25] The primary goal of nonsurgical treatment is relief from symptoms that may be related to inflammation, training errors, limb alignment, flexibility, and muscle weakness. Although many nonsurgical options are available, including activity modification, orthotics, stretching and strengthening exercises, nonsteroidal anti-inflammatory drugs, few have been tested under controlled conditions. Newer nonsurgical methods, such as extracorporeal shock wave therapy (ESWT), sclerosing therapy, electrocoagulation, topical glyceryl trinitrate (GTN), and low-level laser therapy, are currently being investigated and are described elsewhere in this issue. Alfredson and Cook[26] included several of these interventions in their suggested treatment algorithm, recommending surgical treatment only after a lengthy trial of several nonsurgical treatment methods (**Fig. 3**).

Peritendinous injection of a local anesthetic (lidocaine or bupivacaine), a technique called brisement, may help to break up adhesions between the mesotendon and the tendon. Ultrasound guidance can be used to ensure proper placement of the needle. Approximately 5 to 10 mL of the dilute local anesthetic are slowly injected into the paratenon sheath. In about 50% of patients, 2 or 3 injections are successful in decreasing symptoms, especially those with audible crepitus with ambulation.[3,16,27]

SURGICAL TREATMENT

Surgical interventions for the treatment of Achilles tendinopathy include percutaneous longitudinal tenotomies, excision of the degenerated area of the tendon, and augmentation of the debrided tendon segment, usually with the flexor hallucis longus tendon. Surgical intervention is indicated when nonsurgical methods fail to relieve symptoms; factors such as increased patient age, prolonged duration of symptoms, and presence of intrasubstance Achilles tendinopathy are also considerations.[28–30] Outcomes of

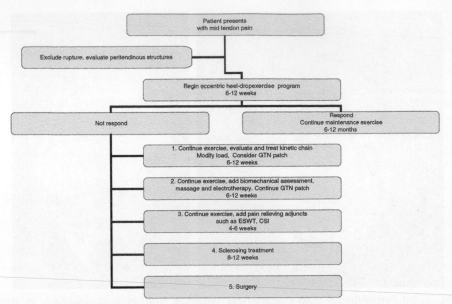

Fig. 3. Suggested algorithm for treatment of patients with Achilles tendinopathy. GTN, glyceryl trinitrate; ESWT, extracorporeal shock-wave therapy; CSI, corticosteroid injections. (*From* Alfredson H, Cook J. A treatment algorithm for managing Achilles tendinopathy: new treatment options. Br J Sports Med 2007;41:211–6; with permission.)

surgical treatment have been shown to be better in athletes than in nonathletes and worse in women than in men.[31] Contraindications to surgery include arterial insufficiency, active skin infection, poor soft-tissue envelope, and medical comorbidities that may increase the risk of surgical complications.

Percutaneous Longitudinal Tenotomy

Percutaneous longitudinal tenotomy is indicated for mild-to-moderate, focal, non-insertional Achilles tendinopathy,[29] especially in patients who are at risk of wound complications. Testa and colleagues[32,33] described a technique of percutaneous longitudinal tenotomy in which multiple, ultrasound-guided, percutaneous incisions are made through the diseased areas of the Achilles tendon. They described their results in 3 series that included 153 athletes: 85 (56%) excellent results, 35 (23%) good results, 20 (13%) fair results, and 13 (8%) poor results.[32–34] According to these investigators, percutaneous tenotomy is simple, can be performed as an outpatient procedure, requires minimal follow-up care, and has few complications.

With the patient prone, the diseased segment of the tendon is identified by palpation or ultrasound, and the area of maximal swelling or tenderness is marked with an indelible pen before administration of the local anesthetic. With a number 11 scalpel blade, a longitudinal stab incision is made parallel to the long axis of the tendon fibers in the marked area. With the cutting edge of the scalpel pointing proximally, the ankle is fully dorsiflexed; then, with the cutting edge pointing distally, the ankle is fully plantar flexed. This is repeated through 4 more separate stab incisions, approximately 2 cm apart: 1 medial and proximal, 1 medial and distal, 1 lateral and proximal, and 1 lateral and distal. The stab incisions are closed with adhesive strips. Early active dorsiflexion and plantar flexion are encouraged, and full weight-bearing generally is allowed 2 or 3 days after surgery, at which time isometric, concentric, and eccentric strengthening exercises are begun. Return to full activity usually is possible at 4 to 6 weeks after surgery.

Minimally Invasive Tendon Stripping

Based on the precept that the process of neovascularization in the damaged tendon is the source of the patient's pain, Longo and colleagues[35] described a minimally invasive technique for tendon stripping as a treatment for Achilles tendinopathy. In their technique, four 0.5-cm longitudinal skin incisions are made: 2 just medial and lateral to the origin of the tendon and 2 just medial and lateral to the distal end of the tendon close to its insertion. A mosquito hemostat is inserted in the incisions, and the proximal and distal portions of Achilles tendon are freed of all the peritendinous adhesions. A number 1 unmounted Ethibond (Ethicon, Somerville, NJ, USA) suture thread is inserted proximally, passing through the 2 proximal incisions over the anterior aspect of the Achilles tendon. The Ethibond is retrieved from the distal incisions over the deep aspect of the Achilles tendon. The Ethibond is slid onto the tendon, causing it to be stripped and freed from adhesions. The procedure is repeated for the superficial aspect of the Achilles tendon. Longitudinal percutaneous tenotomies parallel to the tendon fibers are done, if necessary. According to the investigators, this technique has the advantage of achieving a safe and secure disruption of neovessels and the accompanying nerve supply in a minimally invasive fashion; however, no clinical results were reported.

Endoscopic Tendon Debridement

In an attempt to decrease postoperative complications and speed up return to activity, several investigators have described endoscopic techniques for tendon debridement.[36–39] An arthroscopic shaver is used to release the tendon and to debride the peritenon. Although excellent results have been reported with this technique, most series are small and the follow-up is short. Steenstra and van Dijk[37] reported endoscopic release in 20 successive patients, all of whom had significant pain relief at follow-up of 2 to 7 years (average 6 years); most were able to resume sports activities in 4 to 6 weeks.

Open Tendon Debridement and Repair, with or without Augmentation

For moderate-to-severe tendinopathy (**Fig. 4**A), an open procedure generally is required. The success of open debridement seems to be related to the duration of symptoms, with better outcomes in those with shorter symptom duration.[25,29,40] Peritendinous adhesions also have been implicated as factors producing less favorable results,[24] and release or excision of the constricting paratenon improves results.[41]

Through an approximately 10-cm incision centered over the diseased section of the tendon, the paratenon is carefully incised and any inflammatory peritendinitis is removed with a rongeur. The medial border of the tendon is retracted to allow access to the deep involved portion of the tendon, and the area is debrided sharply until normal tendon is established (**Fig. 4**B). Removal of all the diseased tendon is essential, because any residual degenerated tissue increases the risk of persistent postoperative pain.[29,42]

If more than 50% of the tendon is involved, the flexor hallucis longus (FHL) is transferred to augment the debrided Achilles tendon (**Fig. 4**C).[43] The FHL can be harvested through the same posterior approach to the Achilles tendon used for the debridement; however, a cadaver study has suggested that a more distal FHL harvest through a second, more distal incision provides an average of 3 cm more of FHL tendon

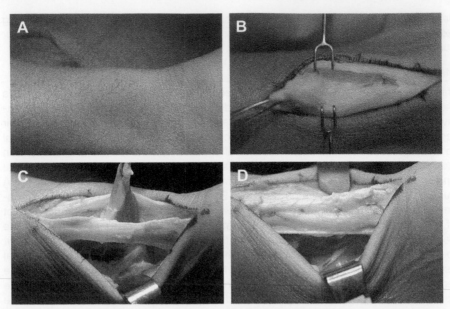

Fig. 4. Open Achilles debridement with FHL transfer. (*A*) Clinical appearance before surgery (same patient as in 2B). (*B*) Debridement of degenerative tendon. (*C*) Transfer of FHL harvested from posterior subtalar level. (*D*) FHL sutured in place. Patient resumed running competitively 5 months after surgery.

length.[44] With the single-incision harvest, the tibial nerve is at risk, whereas with the two-incision harvest the tibial and plantar nerves are at risk. Den Hartog[42] recommended avoiding a second midfoot incision because the extra tendon length is not needed and the extra incision increases surgical time, risk, and morbidity.

The FHL muscle belly and tendon are sewn into the defect created by the debridement, and the tendon is passed through a tunnel drilled from medial to lateral in the calcaneal tuberosity. The FHL tendon is secured with sutures or with an interference-type absorbable screw in the bone tunnel. For non-insertional tendinitis, if the insertion is not debrided and less than 75% of the proximal diseased tendon is removed, no bone fixation is required (**Fig. 4**D).

Most reports indicate good-to-excellent results in 75% to 100% of patients after open debridement procedures.[5,12,34] Maffulli and colleagues,[45] however, reported that only 5 of 14 athletes had good results after open debridement procedures.

Will and Galey[46] reported single-incision FHL transfer in 19 patients, with excellent clinical outcomes and no complications. Using a two-incision technique, Wilcox and colleagues[47] obtained American Orthopaedic Foot and Ankle Society scores of 70 or higher in 18 (90%) of 20 patients. Reported complications of FHL transfer for Achilles tendinopathy include persistent pain and swelling in the tendon, skin necrosis, and rupture of the transferred tendon. Weakness of the hallux at the interphalangeal joint can result from this transfer, but this does not appear to cause any patient discomfort or dysfunction.[43]

SUMMARY

Although excellent results can be obtained with surgical treatment, approximately 20% of patients will require reoperation, and 3% to 5% of patients give up their athletic careers because of persistent Achilles tendon pain.[48] Surgical treatment also is not without complications.[24,49,50] Paavola and colleagues[24] documented an 11% complication rate in 432 consecutive patients who were treated surgically for Achilles tendinopathy. These complications included skin edge necrosis (14), superficial wound infections (11), seroma formation (5), hematoma (5), fibrotic reaction or scar formation (5), sural nerve irritations (4), partial tendon rupture (1), and deep vein thrombosis (1). Most patients who had a complication healed and returned to their preinjury levels of activity, but the frequency of complications should remind the surgeon that surgical treatment should be chosen carefully and individualized to the patient's age, activity level, duration of symptoms, and severity of tendon involvement.

REFERENCES

1. Aström M. Laser Doppler flowmetry in the assessment of tendon blood flow. Scand J Med Sci Sports 2000;10:365–7.
2. Movin T, Kristoffersen-Wiberg M, Shalabi A, et al. Intraintendinous alterations as imaged by ultrasound and contrast-enhanced magnetic resonance in chronic achillodynia. Foot Ankle Int 1998;19:311–7.
3. Reddy SS, Pedowitz DI, Parekh SG, et al. Surgical treatment for chronic disease and disorders of the Achilles tendon. J Am Acad Orthop Surg 2009;17:3–14.
4. Rees JD, Maffulli N, Cook J. Management of tendinopathy. Am J Sports Med 2009 [Epub ahead of print.]
5. Maffulli N, Kader D. Tendinopathy of tendo achillis. J Bone Joint Surg Br 2002;84: 1–8.
6. Maffulli N, Kahn KM. Clinical nomenclature for tendon injuries. Med Sci Sports Exerc 1999;31:352–3.
7. Clancy WG Jr, Neidhart D, Brand RL. Achilles tendonitis in runners: a report of five cases. Am J Sports Med 1976;4:46–57.
8. Clain MR, Baxter DE. Achilles tendinitis. Foot Ankle 1992;13:482–7.
9. Puddu G, Ippolito E, Postachini F. A classification of Achilles tendon disease. Am J Sports Med 1976;4:145–50.
10. de Mos M, van El B, DeGroot J, et al. Achilles tendinosis: changes in biochemical composition and collagen turnover rate. Am J Sports Med 2007;35:1549–56.
11. McShane JM, Ostick B, McCabe F. Noninsertional Achilles tendinopathy: pathology and management. Curr Sports Med Rep 2007;6:288–92.
12. Rolf C, Movin T. Etiology, histopathology, and outcome of surgery in achillodynia. Foot Ankle Int 1997;18:565–9.
13. Alfredson H. The chronic painful Achilles and patellar tendon: research on basic biology and treatment. Scand J Med Sci Sports 2005;15:252–9.
14. Alfredson H, Thorsen K, Lorentzon R. In situ microdialysis in tendon tissue: high levels of glutamate, but not prostaglandin E2 in chronic Achilles tendon pain. Knee Surg Sports Traumatol Arthrosc 1999;7:378–81.
15. Schubert TE, Weidler C, Lerch K, et al. Achilles tendinosis is associated with sprouting of substance P positive nerve fibres. Ann Rheum Dis 2005;64:1083–6.
16. Saltzman CL, Tearse DS. Achilles tendon injuries. J Am Acad Orthop Surg 1998; 6:316–25.
17. Strocchi R, De Pasquale V, Guizzardi S, et al. Human Achilles tendon: morphological and morphometric variations as a function of age. Foot Ankle 1991;12:100–4.
18. Raleigh SM, van der Merwe L, Ribbans WJ, et al. Variants within the MMP3 gene are associated with Achilles tendinopathy: possible interaction with the COL5A1 gene. Br J Sports Med 2009;43:514–20.

19. O'Brien M. The anatomy of the Achilles tendon. Foot Ankle Clin 2005;10:225–38.
20. Carr AJ, Norris SH. The blood supply of the calcaneal tendon. J Bone Joint Surg Br 1989;71:100–1.
21. Kvist M, Hurme T, Kannus P, et al. Vascular density at the myotendinous junction of the rate gastrocnemius muscle after immobilization and remobilization. Am J Sports Med 1995;23:359–64.
22. Lagergren C, Lindholm A. Vascular distribution in the Achilles tendon: an angiographic and microangiographic study. Acta Chir Scand 1959;116:491–5.
23. Magnussen RA, Dunn WR, Thomson AB. Nonoperative treatment of midportion Achilles tendinopathy: a systematic review. Clin J Sport Med 2009;19:54–64.
24. Paavola M, Kannus P, Paakkala T, et al. Long-term prognosis of patients with Achilles tendinopathy. An observational 8-year follow-up study. Am J Sports med 2000;28:634–42.
25. Johnston E, Scranton P Jr, Pfeffer GB. Chronic disorders of the Achilles tendon: results of conservative and surgical treatments. Foot Ankle 1997;18:570–4.
26. Alfredson H, Cook J. A treatment algorithm for managing Achilles tendinopathy: new treatment options. Br J Sports Med 2007;41:211–6.
27. Schepsis AA, Jones H, Maas AL. Achilles tendon disorders in athletes. Am J Sports Med 2002;30:287–305.
28. Rompe JD, Furia JP, Maffulli N. Mid-portion Achilles tendinopathy—current options for treatment. Disabil Rehabil 2008;30:20–2.
29. Scott A, Kahn K. Tendon overuse pathology: implications for clinical management. In: Kibler WB, editor. Orthopaedic knowledge update 4: sports medicine. Rosemont (IL): American Academy of Orthopaedic Surgeons; 2009. p. 307–42.
30. Scott AT, Le IL, Easley ME. Surgical strategies: non-insertional Achilles tendinopathy. Foot Ankle Int 2008;29:759–71.
31. Maffulli N, Testa V, Capasso G, et al. Surgery for chronic Achilles tendinopathy produces worse results in women. Disabil Rehabil 2008;30:1714–20.
32. Testa V, Capasso G, Benazzo F, et al. Management of Achilles tendinopathy by ultrasound-guided percutaneous tenotomy. Med Sci Sports Exerc 2002;34:573–80.
33. Testa V, Maffulli N, Capasso G, et al. Percutaneous longitudinal tenotomy in chronic Achilles tendonitis. Bull Hosp Jt Dis 1996;54:241–4.
34. Maffulli N, Testa V, Capasso G, et al. Results of percutaneous longitudinal tenotomy for Achilles tendinopathy in middle- and long-distance runners. Am J Sports Med 1997;25:835–40.
35. Longo UG, Ramamurthy C, Denaro V, et al. Minimally invasive stripping for chronic Achilles tendinopathy. Disabil Rehabil 2008;30:1709–13.
36. Maquirriain J, Ayerza M, Costa-Pas M, et al. Endoscopic surgery in chronic Achilles tendinopathies: a preliminary report. Arthroscopy 2002;18:298–303.
37. Steenstra F, van Dijk CN. Achilles tendoscopy. Foot Ankle Clin 2006;11:429–38.
38. Thermann H, Benetos IS, Panelli C, et al. Endoscopic treatment of chronic mid-portion Achilles tendinopathy: novel technique with short-term results. Knee Surg Sports Traumatol Arthrosc 2009 [Epub ahead of print.]
39. Vega J, Cabestany JM, Golanó P, et al. Endoscopic treatment for chronic Achilles tendinopathy. Foot Ankle Surg 2008;14:204–10.
40. Benazzo F, Stennardo G, Valli M. Achilles and patellar tendinopathies in athletes: pathogenesis and surgical treatment. Bull Hosp Jt Dis 1996;54:236–40.
41. Gould N, Korson R. Stenosing tenosynovitis of the pseudosheath of the tendo Achilles. Foot Ankle 1980;1:179–87.

42. Den Hartog BD. Midsubstance Achilles Tendinopathy. AAOS orthopaedic knowledge online. Available at: www5.aaos.org/oko. Accessed May 8, 2009.
43. Den Hartog BD. Flexor hallucis longus transfer for chronic Achilles tendinosis. Foot Ankle Int 2003;24:233–7.
44. Tashjian RZ, Hur J, Sullivan RJ, et al. Flexor hallucis longus transfer for repair of chronic achilles tendinopathy. Foot Ankle Int 2003;24:673–6.
45. Maffulli N, Binfield PM, Moore D, et al. Surgical decompression of chronic central core lesions of the Achilles tendon. Am J Sports Med 1999;27:747–52.
46. Will RE, Galey SM. Outcome of single incision flexor hallucis longus transfer for chronic Achilles tendinopathy. Foot Ankle Int 2009;30:315–7.
47. Wilcox DK, Bohay DR, Anderson JB. Treatment of chronic Achilles tendon disorders with flexor hallucis longus tendon transfer/augmentation. Foot Ankle Int 2007;28:149–53.
48. Alfredson H, Lorentzon R. Chronic Achilles tendinosis: recommendations for treatment and prevention. Sports Med 2000;29:135–46.
49. Mulier T, Rummens E, Dereymaeker G. Risk of neurovascular injuries in flexor hallucis tendon transfers: an anatomic cadaver study. Foot Ankle Int 2007;28:910–5.
50. Saxena A, Maffulli N, Nguyen A, et al. Wound complications from surgeries pertaining to the Achilles tendon: an analysis of 219 surgeries. J Am Podiatr Med Assoc 2008;98:95–101.

Conservative Treatment of Achilles Tendinopathy: Emerging Techniques

Jason E. Lake, MD[a], Susan N. Ishikawa, MD[b],*

KEYWORDS

• Achilles tendon • Tendinopathy • Achilles tendinosis
• Achilles pain • Nonsurgical treatment

Achilles tendinopathy, a painful condition that can be acute or chronic, is common in both active and inactive individuals.[1–8] Pain may be present in the mid-substance or at the tendon's insertion, and swelling of the tendon may be noted. The diagnosis of Achilles tendinopathy usually is made clinically, but ultrasound or MRI can be used to assist in the diagnosis or rule out other pathology in the region.[9–11] Differential diagnoses include os trigonum syndrome; peroneal tendon disorders; stress fractures of the ankle or hindfoot; plantar flexor tenosynovitis; an accessory soleus muscle; tumor of the Achilles tendon (xanthoma); sural neuroma; and peritendinopathy.[12] This article focuses on newer nonsurgical methods of treatment of mid-substance Achilles tendinopathy.

PATHOPHYSIOLOGY

A number of possible etiologies have been suggested for Achilles tendinopathy, including overuse (although tendinopathy also occurs in inactive individuals); decreased blood supply and tensile strength with aging; muscle imbalance or weakness; insufficient flexibility; or malalignment (hyperpronation).[6,7,12–19] Most of these theories are based on poor scientific evidence. Biopsies of affected Achilles tendons reveal cellular activation and increases in cell numbers and ground substance, collagen disarray, and neovascularization.[1] Prostaglandin inflammatory elements are not present, but neurogenic inflammatory elements, such as substance P and calcitonin gene-related peptide, have been isolated.[17,20–24] Neurovascular ingrowth

[a] Campbell Clinic, University of Tennessee, 1211 Union Avenue, Suite 510, Memphis, TN 38104, USA
[b] Campbell Clinic, University of Tennessee, 1458 West Poplar Avenue, Suite 100, Collierville, TN 38017, USA
* Corresponding author.
E-mail address: sishikawa@campbellclinic.com (S.N. Ishikawa).

Foot Ankle Clin N Am 14 (2009) 663–674
doi:10.1016/j.fcl.2009.07.003
1083-7515/09/$ – see front matter © 2009 Elsevier Inc. All rights reserved.

foot.theclinics.com

and glutamate (a potent modulator of pain) have been noted in diseased tendons and have been postulated to be the source of pain in patients with Achilles tendinopathy.[25,26]

CONSERVATIVE TREATMENT METHODS
Traditional Noninvasive Methods

Initial treatment usually begins with traditional noninvasive measures that include activity modification; orthotics (to correct malalignment); stretching; heel lifts to reduce tension in the tendon; massage; heat and cold therapy; traditional strengthening exercises; ultrasound; and nonsteroidal anti-inflammatory drugs or oral corticosteroids.[1,3,4,6,12,15,16,18,19] The use of nonsteroidal anti-inflammatory drugs has been questioned because of the absence of evidence of prostaglandin inflammatory mediators within the diseased tendon.[27] In a randomized, double-blind, placebo-controlled trial, oral piroxicam was no more effective than placebo.[28] Generally favorable outcomes have been reported for traditional noninvasive methods, but in about 30% of patients these are ineffective.[29] As a result, other modalities have been investigated.

Corticosteroid Injection

Although corticosteroid injections are commonly used for other tendinopathies, their role in Achilles tendinopathy has yet to be established. Short-term pain relief was reported after peritendinous corticosteroid injections in one randomized controlled trial,[30] but another demonstrated no improvement.[31] Although intratendinous injections have been discouraged by some authors, others have recommended intratendinous injections.[32,33] In a case series of peritendinous corticosteroid injections reported by Gill and colleagues,[34] there were no tendon ruptures, but only 40% of patients reported improvement. Currently, there are no well-designed, randomized, prospective, clinical trials documenting the efficacy of corticosteroid injections. Given the lack of published data regarding corticosteroid benefits and the multiple reports of Achilles tendon complete or partial ruptures after corticosteroid injection, the authors are very cautious regarding their use at this time.[35–38]

Eccentric Training

In the 1980s, Stanish and coworkers[39] emphasized the importance of an eccentric training program in the treatment of tendon injuries. Alfredson and colleagues[40] later adapted this program for painful mid-substance Achilles tendinopathy. This exercise program does not involve any concentric loading, exercises are performed even if pain is present, and load is increased until pain is present. In multiple studies, this 12-week program has produced good results in up to 90% of patients with mid-substance tendinopathy, but in only approximately 30% of those with insertional Achilles tendinopathy.[35,40–44] A recent randomized controlled trial comparing extracorporeal shockwave therapy (ESWT) with eccentric training and placebo by Rompe and colleagues[35] reported a 60% success rate with the eccentric loading program in patients with noninsertional tendinopathy. Another randomized controlled trial by Rompe and colleagues[41] comparing the same treatment modalities, but in patients with insertional Achilles tendinopathy, supported data by Fahlstrom and colleagues[42] showing poor success (28%) with eccentric loading in this group.

Several theories have been proposed to explain the effectiveness of eccentric exercise (EE) in reducing mid-substance Achilles tendon pain. Short-term effects include increased tendon volume and signal intensity, which is thought to be a response to trauma and may promote healing of the tendon[45]; however, after a 12-week program, a decrease in size and a more normal tendon appearance were noted on ultrasound and MRI.[46–48] Some believe that eccentric loading may lengthen the muscle-tendon unit over time and increase its capacity to bear load. Also, because vessels disappear on imaging with muscle contraction and stretch, repetitive eccentric training may damage abnormal vessels and accompanying nerves in this region of the tendon.[1,49]

Extracorporeal Shock Wave Therapy

ESWT has been shown to stimulate angiogenesis and inhibit afferent pain receptor function and may improve soft tissue healing.[50,51] It also has been shown to produce a higher number of neovessels and markers, such as nitric oxide synthase (NOS).[26,52–54] Shock wave therapy can be given in a low-energy or high-energy form. The low-energy treatment does not require local or intravenous anesthesia and usually is given in three weekly sessions. High-energy ESWT is given in one session but requires local or intravenous anesthesia.[55,56]

Since the late 1980s ESWT has been used successfully to treat such disorders as plantar fasciitis, shoulder calcific tendonitis, and lateral epicondylitis.[55,56] More recently, several studies have reported successful ESWT treatment of Achilles tendinopathy.[35,41,55,56] In two nonrandomized clinical trials, Furia[55,56] reported that the percentages of successful results 12 months after treatment of both noninsertional and insertional Achilles tendinopathy were statistically greater in patients treated with high-energy ESWT than in those treated with traditional nonoperative methods. Additionally, in a randomized, double-blind, placebo controlled trial with 39 patients, Peers[57] reported a significant improvement in the visual analog scores of patients treated with low energy ESWT compared with untreated patients.

In a randomized controlled trial of patients with noninsertional tendinosis, Rompe and colleagues[35] compared eccentric loading, low-energy ESWT, and a wait-and-see policy in groups of 25 patients each. At 4-month follow-up, eccentric and low-energy ESWT had comparable results and were superior (50%–60% success rates) to the wait-and-see policy (24% success rate). A similar study by Rompe and colleagues[41] showed low-energy ESWT to be superior to eccentric loading for insertional Achilles tendinopathy.

Costa and colleagues,[58] in a double-blind, randomized, placebo-controlled trial involving 49 patients, found no difference between high-energy ESWT and the control group. Because the protocol in this study was different from that in previous studies, however, and the study groups were small (possible type II error), the results of the study have been questioned.[59]

Although not widely available, ESWT does seem to be beneficial in level I studies and may have a place in future management of Achilles tendinopathy.

Sclerosing Agents

Sclerosing therapy for chronic Achilles tendinosis is based on the premise that the process of neovascularization in the damaged tendon is the source of the patient's pain. Studies in the European literature have implicated neurovascularization as possible pain generators in Achilles tendinopathy, possibly because of the sensory nerves linked to the vessels, and these findings led to the hypothesis that destruction of the vessels and nerves leads to pain relief.

In a pilot study published in 2002, Ohberg and Alfredson[60] reported the use of polidocanol (Kreussler, Wiesbaden, Germany) as a sclerosing agent for the treatment of Achilles tendinopathy. Polidocanol (first developed as a local anesthetic) results in thrombosis through a selective effect on the intima, and this occurs even when the drug is injected extravascularly. This extravascular effect is important when the drug is used for sclerosing the very small neovessels surrounding an injured Achilles tendon, because intravascular injection is not practical in this location. Extravascular injection also may have a destructive or ischemic effect on adjacent nerves, which can help with pain modulation.[61]

Currently, almost all the reports of sclerosing therapy with polidocanol are from one institution in Sweden and most are retrospective case series with relatively short follow-up. In one small double-blind study, 20 consecutive patients were randomized to receive polidocanol injection just outside the ventral part of the tendon where neovessels were present or lidocaine with adrenaline injection localized with color Doppler ultrasound. At 3-month follow-up, after a maximum of two treatments 3 and 6 weeks apart, 5 of the 10 patients receiving the sclerosing agent were satisfied and had a significantly reduced amount of tendon pain. None of the control group was satisfied. After patients in the lidocaine group were treated with the sclerosing agent, 9 of 10 were satisfied, giving a 70% (14 of 20) overall success rate.[61] Although the authors did not evaluate the tendons for neovascularization at follow-up, in a previous pilot study by the same authors, tendons that were pain-free did not have neovascularization inside or outside of the tendon.[48,61] The promising short-term results led to a longer-term study at the same institution involving 42 patients, all treated with sclerosing therapy. At 2-year follow-up, 37 (88%) patients were satisfied with their results and had returned to preinjury activity levels. Color Doppler ultrasound evaluation showed a significant reduction in tendon thickness and significantly fewer neovessels.[62] Alfredson and colleagues[63] later compared polidocanol injection with open surgical revision of the area of neural and vascular ingrowth in the ventral side of the tendon. At 6-month follow-up, six of nine patients who had ultrasound-guided injections were satisfied and all 10 patients who had ultrasound-guided surgery were satisfied.

No serious adverse events were noted in these studies, though Alfredson and Cook[1] did report one rupture and one partial rupture out of the 400 tendons treated with sclerosing therapy. The usual protocol is two or three sclerosing injections given approximately 6 to 8 weeks apart. Each injection is followed by a few days of rest and high-impact activity is restricted for 2 weeks. As a result, treatment with sclerosing agents can be a long process; however, with its relatively high success rate and low complication rate, sclerosing therapy may be a viable treatment option for those in whom more conservative measures are unsuccessful.

Electrocoagulation

Given the success of sclerosing therapy, Boesen and colleagues[64] evaluated ultrasound-guided electrocoagulation in 11 patients with chronic mid-portion tendinopathy. This was performed as an office procedure under local anesthesia. The electrocautery needle was introduced percutaneously and used to cauterize the neovessels on the anterior aspect of the tendon after localization of the vessels with ultrasound. Ten of the 11 patients had Likert pain scores (0–10) reduced from a median of 7 to 0 at 6-month follow-up after one treatment. Color Doppler ultrasound, however, noted a return of neovessels at 2 weeks after treatment. The authors postulated that the pain relief was a result of nerve destruction and unrelated to changes in blood flow.

Topical Glyceryl Trinitrate

Topical glyceryl trinitrate (GTN) is a prodrug of endogenous nitric oxide and is commercially available as a topical patch to deliver nitric oxide, which is a soluble gas that acts as a messenger molecule that can affect many cellular functions, including tendon healing.[65,66] Suggested mechanisms for the effects of nitric oxide on tendon healing have included an increase in collagen production by fibroblasts, an increase in cellular adhesion, and an increase in local vascularity.[67–71] In a rat Achilles tendon healing model, Murrell and colleagues[72] noted a fivefold increase in NOS that peaked at day 7. This increase in NOS also was noted in injured and over-used rat rotator cuff tendons.[67,73] Rats taking NOS inhibitor had reduced healing with 50% reduction in cross-sectional area of the Achilles tendon on day 7.[72] In random-ized, double-blind, placebo-controlled trials, Paoloni and colleagues[74] reported similar findings in humans with Achilles tendinopathy, tennis elbow, and chronic supraspinatus tendinopathy. In the Achilles tendon study, 27 (78%) of 36 tendons treated with 1.25 mg topical GTN every 24 hours for 6 months had excellent results, whereas only 20 (49%) of 41 in the placebo group had excellent results. Both groups also were treated with concurrent rest, heel wedges, and stretching followed by eccentric strengthening. A follow-up by the same authors on the same group of patients noted that 88% of GTN patients and 67% of placebo patients were completely asymptomatic at 3 years.[75] The most common side effects of GTN included headaches and a rash at the site of patch application, although there was no significant difference in the incidence when compared with the placebo group.[74,75]

More recently, Kane and colleagues[71] compared topical GTN with standard phys-ical therapy in 40 patients with noninsertional Achilles tendinopathy. After 6 months of treatment, there were no significant differences in Ankle Osteoarthritis Scale visual analog score for pain or disability between the two groups. Additionally, patients who failed treatment at 6 months were treated with surgical decompression and had histo-logic samples taken. Histologic and immunohistochemical examinations found no differences in neovascularization, collagen synthesis, or stimulated fibroblasts between the two groups. No evidence of modulation of NOS was noted.

Although there seems to be evidence at the cellular level of the role of nitric oxide in tendon healing, there have been some conflicting clinical studies in human Achilles tendons suggesting that further validation is needed before it can be recommended for widespread use.

Aprotinin Injections

Several studies have demonstrated an increase in matrix metalloproteinases in tendin-opathy, specifically the collagenases and gelatinases.[76–79] Because the presence of excess collagenases may play an important role in tendinopathy, aprotinin, a serine protease inhibitor (particularly plasmin) and a strong inhibitor of matrix metalloprotei-nases, has been suggested as a treatment. Treatment of Achilles tendinopathy with aprotinin involves a peritendinous injection that can be done in the office.[80–89] Used since the 1960s to help prevent blood loss and promote healing, aprotinin is a compo-nent of fibrin glue.[84,86]

Uncontrolled studies of the use of aprotinin in the treatment of Achilles tendinopathy have produced approximately 80% success rates.[80,85] Capasso and colleagues,[81] in a semi-randomized study, noted a prompt return to play in 78% of patients treated with aprotinin compared with 30% of the placebo group. In a randomized controlled trial (33 tendons total), Brown and colleagues[87] compared aprotinin injections (one per week for 3 weeks) with normal saline injections (placebo). Both groups partici-pated in an eccentric training program. At no follow-up point (2, 4, 12, or 52 weeks) was there any statistically significant difference between the groups. Orchard and colleagues[84] published a large, retrospective, case-series of 343 patients (from the same institution as Brown and colleagues[87]) who completed questionnaires at follow-up ranging from 3 to 54 months (average, 12 months); 84% of those with mid-Achilles tendinopathy and 69% of those with insertional Achilles tendinopathy thought aprotinin injections were helpful. The level of evidence is low in this study, however, given its retrospective nature, lack of a control group, and the fact that many additional treatments were used.

Risks are present with aprotinin injections, mainly allergic reactions ranging from itching to anaphylaxis (3%–11%).[84,87–89] Brown and colleagues[87] reported the rate of itching as about 25% and the rate of systemic reaction as about 7% per patient (2.5% per injection). Orchard and colleagues[84] stated that true anaphylactic reaction is probably less than 1% but greater than 0.1% as previously published. Because the reaction occurs through immunologic mechanisms, especially with multiple frequent dosing, Orchard and colleagues[89] recommended a one-time dose or a delay of at least 6 weeks between dosing to lower the risk of severe allergic reaction. Additionally, as of November 2007, Bayer has temporarily suspended sales of aprotinin for reasons unrelated to its use for treatment of tendinopathy.

Given its risk profile and the lack of level I evidence documenting its efficacy, aprotinin needs to be further evaluated with prospective, randomized, controlled studies (if it becomes available at a later date) before it can be recommended.

Low-level Laser Therapy

Low-level laser therapy (LLLT) has been used for many years in the treatment of several disorders, including rheumatoid disorders, low back pain, and osteoarthritis.[90] LLLT may stimulate both acute anti-inflammatory and regenerative processes and has been shown to reduce cell apoptosis and promote collagen fiber synthesis.[90–92] It has been shown that LLLT has a dose-dependent (2–10 J/cm^2) and wavelength-dependent (810–830 nm) therapeutic window.[90]

In a randomized controlled trial, Stergioulas and colleagues[90] compared EE with EE and LLLT in 52 patients. In addition to EE, patients in the LLLT group received LLLT in 12 sessions over 8 weeks in which six points along the mid-substance of the diseased Achilles tendon were irradiated. Pain intensity during physical activity on a 100-mm visual analog scale was significantly less in the EE plus LLLT group (53.6 mm) compared with the EE alone group (71.5 mm). This trend continued at 12 weeks. Additionally, morning stiffness, tenderness to palpation, active dorsiflexion, and crepitus also were significantly improved. There were no significant side effects.

Although LLLT seems to be safe, there have been few studies regarding its use to treat the Achilles tendon, and results of these studies need to be verified with further research before LLLT becomes a standard treatment option.

OTHER TREATMENTS

Several other treatment methods have been investigated, but few well-designed studies are available for review. Prolotherapy, which involves the injection of hyperosmolar dextrose to act as an irritant that initiates an inflammatory response and presumably healing, has been reported to be successful in the treatment of chronic Achilles tendinosis by Maxwell and colleagues.[93] At 6-month follow-up after this treatment, 20 of 30 patients were asymptomatic, nine had mild symptoms, and one had moderate symptoms. Similarly, autologous blood injections have been used clinically with promising results (G.A. Murphy, personal communication, 2009). This has been tried given its success in the treatment of lateral epicondylitis,[94,95] medial epicondylitis,[96] patellar tendinosis,[97] and plantar fasciitis.[98] Giombini and colleagues[99] reported success with hyperthermia and low-frequency microwave treatment. In another study,

2 weeks of microcurrent, which is similar to transcutaneous electrical nerve stimulation but with lower amperage that is theoretically more physiologic, has been shown to decrease pain at 12-month follow-up.[100] Platelet-rich plasma injections have been evaluated in the healing of ruptured tendons but not tendinopathy.[101,102] Additionally, BMP-12 and BMP-14 gene therapy is being studied in rat models but not in human Achilles tendons to date.[103,104]

SUMMARY

Achilles tendinopathy is a common disorder, but the pathology is still not completely understood. For example, some treatment methods are reported to be effective because they increase neovessel formation, whereas other emerging treatments aim to reduce the number of neovessels. Nonetheless, most patients find relief with traditional conservative treatments. The subset of patients with persistent symptoms is the target of these emerging techniques. With the exception of EE, which are noninvasive, low-cost, and readily available, further prospective studies are needed to demonstrate clinical efficacy and cost effectiveness of other nonoperative treatment methods.

REFERENCES

1. Alfredson H, Cook J. A treatment algorithm for managing Achilles tendinopathy: new treatment options. Br J Sports Med 2007;41:211–6.
2. Myerson M, McGarvey W. Disorders of the Achilles insertion and Achilles tendonitis. Instr Course Lect 1999;48:211–8.
3. Kvist M. Achilles tendon injuries in athletes. Sports Med 1994;18(3):173–201.
4. Curvin S, Standish WD. Tendinitis: its etiology and treatment. Lexington (KY): Collamore Press, DC Heath & Co.; 1984.
5. Archambault JM, Wiley P, Bay RC. Exercise loading of tendons and the development of overuse injuries: a review. Sports Med 1995;20(2):77–89.
6. Jozsa LG, Kannus P. Human tendons: anatomy, physiology, and pathology. Champaign (IL): Human Kinetics Publishers; 1997. p. 1–573.
7. Movin T. Aspects of aetiology, pathoanatomy and diagnostic methods in chronic mid-portion Achillodynia [doctoral dissertation]. Stockholm (Sweden): Karolinska Institute Stockholm; 1998.
8. Alfredson H, Lorentzon R. Chronic Achilles tendinosis: recommendations for treatment and prevention. Sports Med 2000;29(2):135–46.
9. Astrom M, Gentz CF, Nilsson P, et al. Imaging in chronic Achilles tendinopathy: a comparison of ultrasonography, magnetic resonance imaging and surgical findings in 27 histologically verified cases. Skeletal Radiol 1996;25:615–20.
10. Paavola M, Paakkala T, Kannus P, et al. Ultrasonography in the differential diagnosis of Achilles tendon injuries and related disorders. Acta Radiol 1998;39: 612–9.
11. Neuhold A, Stiskal M, Kainberger F, et al. Degenerative Achilles tendon disease: assessment by magnetic resonance and ultrasonography. Eur J Radiol 1992;14: 213–20.
12. Alfredson H. Conservative management of Achilles tendinopathy: new ideas. Foot Ankle Clin 2005;10:321–9.
13. Welsh RP, Clodman J. Clinical survey of Achilles tendinitis in athletes. Can Med Assoc J 1980;122:193–5.
14. Astrom M. Partial rupture in Achilles tendinopathy: a retrospective analysis of 342 cases. Acta Orthop Scand 1998;69:404–7.

15. Clement DB, Taunton JE, Smart GW. Achilles tendinitis and peritendinitis: etiology and treatment. Am J Sports Med 1984;12:179–84.
16. Nichols AW. Achilles tendinitis in running athletes. J Am Board Fam Pract 1989; 2:196–203.
17. Maffulli N, Khan KM, Puddu G. Overuse tendon conditions: time to change a confusing terminology. Arthroscopy 1998;14:840–3.
18. James SL, Bates BT, Osternig LR. Injuries to runners. Am J Sports Med 1978; 6(2):40–50.
19. Galloway MT, Jokl P, Dayton OW. Achilles tendon overuse injuries. Clin Sports Med 1992;11(4):771–82.
20. Alfredson H, Forsgren S, Thorsen K, et al. Glutamate NMDAR1 receptors localized to nerves in human Achilles tendons: implications for treatment? Knee Surg Sports Traumatol Arthrosc 2000;9:123–6.
21. Alfredson H, Thorsen K, Lorentzon R. In situ microdialysis in tendon tissue: high levels of glutamate, but not prostoglandin E_2 in chronic Achilles tendon pain. Knee Surg Sports Traumatol Arthrosc 1999;7:378–81.
22. Alfredson H, Lorentzon M, Backman S, et al. cDNA-arrays and real-time quantitative PCR techniques in the investigation of chronic Achilles tendinosis. J Orthop Res 2003;21:970–5.
23. Hart DA, Frank CB, Bray RC. Inflammatory processes in repetitive motion and overuse syndromes: potential role of neurogenic mechanisms in tendons and ligaments. In: Gordon SL, Blair SJ, Fine LJ, editors. Repetitive motion disorders of the upper extremity. Rosemont (IL): American Academy of Orthopaedic Surgeons; 1995. p. 247–62.
24. Scott A, Khan KM, Cook JL, et al. What do we mean by the term "inflammation"? A contemporary basic science update for sports medicine. Br J Sports Med 2004;38:372–80.
25. Alfredson H, Forsgran S, Thorsen K, et al. In vivo microdialysis and immunohistochemical analyses of tendon tissue demonstrated high amounts of free glutamate and glutamate receptors, but no signs of inflammation, in jumpers knee. J Orthop Res 2001;19:881–6.
26. Bjur D, Alfredson H, Forsgren S. The innervation pattern of human Achilles tendon: studies of the normal and tendinosis tendon with markers for general and sensory innervation. Cell Tissue Res 2005;320:201–6.
27. Khan KM, Cook JL, Bonar F, et al. Histopathology of common tendinopatihies: update and implications for clinical management. Sports Med 1999;27(6): 393–408.
28. Astrom M, Westlin N. No effect of piroxicam on Achilles tendinopathy: a randomized study of 70 patients. Acta Orthop Scand 1992;63:631–4.
29. Paavola M, Kannus P, Paakkala T, et al. Long-term prognosis of patients with Achilles tendinopathy: an observational 8-year follow-up study. Am J Sports Med 2000;28:634–42.
30. Smidt N, van der Windt DA, Assendelft W, et al. Corticosteroid injections, physiotherapy, or wait-and-see policy for lateral epicondylitis: a randomized controlled trial. Lancet 2002;359:657–62.
31. Da Cruz DJ, Geeson M, Allen MJ, et al. Achilles paratendonitis: an evaluation of steroid injection. Br J Sports Med 1988;22:64–5.
32. Fredberg U, Bolvig L, Pfeiffer-Jensen M, et al. Ultrasonography as a tool for diagnosis, guidance of local steroid injection and, together with algometry, monitoring of treatment of athletes with chronic jumper's knee and Achilles tendinitis:

a randomized double-blind, placebo-controlled trial. Scand J Rheumatol 2004; 33:94–101.

33. Koenig MJ, Torp-Pederson S, Qvistgaard E, et al. Preliminary results of colour Doppler-guided intratendinous glucocorticoid injection for Achilles tendonitis in five patients. Scand J Med Sci Sports 2004;14(2):100–6.

34. Gill SS, Gelbke MK, Mattson SL, et al. Fluoroscopically guided low-volume peritendinous corticosteroid injection for Achilles tendinopathy. J Bone Joint Surg Am 2004;86(4):802–6.

35. Rompe JD, Nafe B, Furia JP, et al. Eccentric loading, shock-wave treatment, or a wait-and-see policy for tendinopathy of the main body of the tendon Achilles. Am J Sports Med 2007;35:374–83.

36. Kleinman M, Gross AE. Achilles tendon rupture following steroid injection: report of three cases. J Bone Joint Surg Am 1983;65:1345–7.

37. Lee HB. Avulsion and rupture of the tendo calcaneus after injection of hydrocortisone [letter]. BMJ 1957;2:395.

38. Ford LT, DeBender J. Tendon rupture after local steroid injection. Southampt Med J 1979;72:827–30.

39. Stanish WD, Rubinovich RM, Curwin S. Eccentric exercise in chronic tendonitis. Clin Orthop Relat Res 1986;208:65–8.

40. Alfredson H, Pietila T, Jonsson P, et al. Heavy-load eccentric calf muscle training for the treatment of chronic Achilles tendinosis. Am J Sports Med 1998;26: 360–6.

41. Rompe JD, Furia J, Maffulli N. Eccentric loading compared with shock wave treatment for chronic insertional Achilles tendinopathy. J Bone Joint Surg Am 2008;90:52–61.

42. Fahlstrom M, Jonsson P, Lorentzon R, et al. Chronic Achilles tendon pain treated with eccentric calf-muscle training. Knee Surg Sports Traumatol Arthrosc 2003; 11:327–33.

43. Roos E, Engstrom M, Lagerquist A, et al. Clinical improvement after 6 weeks of eccentric exercise in patients with mid-portion Achilles tendinopathy: a randomized trial with 1-year follow-up. Scand J Med Sci Sports 2004;14: 286–95.

44. Fahlstrom M. Badminton and the Achilles tendon [PhD thesis]. Umea, Umea University, 2001.

45. Shalabi A, Kristoffersen-Wilberg M, Aspelin P, et al. Immediate Achilles tendon response after strength training evaluated by MRI. Med Sci Sports Exerc 2004;36:1841–6.

46. Shalabi A, Kristoffersen-Wilberg M, Svensson L, et al. Eccentric training of the gastrocnemius-soleus complex in chronic Achilles tendinopathy results in decreased tendon volume and intratendinous signal as evaluated by MRI. Am J Sports Med 2004;32:1286–96.

47. Ohberg L, Lorentzon R, Alfredson H. Eccentric training in patients with chronic Achilles tendinosis: normalized tendon structure and decreased thickness at follow up. Br J Sports Med 2004;38:8–11.

48. Ohberg L, Lorentzon R, Alfredson H. Neovascularization in Achilles tendons with painful tendinosis but not in normal tendons: an ultrasonographic investigation. Knee Surg Sports Traumatol Arthrosc 2001;9:233–8.

49. Ohberg L, Alfredson H. Effects on neovascularization behind the good results with eccentric training in chronic mid-portion Achilles tendinosis? Knee Surg Sports Traumatol Arthrosc 2004;12:465–70.

50. Takahashi N, Wada Y, Ohtori S, et al. Second application of low-energy shock waves has a cumulative effect on free nerve endings. Clin Orthop Relat Res 2006;443:315–9.
51. Ohtori S, Inoue G, Mannoji C, et al. Shock wave application to rat skin induces degeneration and reinnervation of sensory nerve fibers. Neurosci Lett 2001;315: 57–60.
52. Wang CJ, Huang HY, Pai CH. Shock wave enhances neovasculatization at the tendon-bone junction. J Foot Ankle Surg 2002;41:16–22.
53. Wang CJ, Wang FS, Yang KD, et al. Shock wave therapy induces neovasculatizatin at the tendon-bone junction: a study in rabbits. J Orthop Res 2003;21: 984–9.
54. Chen YJ, Wang CJ, Kuender DY, et al. Extracorporeal shock waves promote healing of collagenase-induced Achilles tendinitis and increase TGF-β1 and IGF-I expression. J Orthop Res 2004;22:854–61.
55. Furia JP. High energy extracorporeal shock wave therapy as a treatment for chronic noninsertional Achilles tendinopathy. Am J Sports Med 2008;36(3): 502–8.
56. Furia JP. High-energy extracorporeal shock wave therapy as treatment for insertional Achilles tendinopathy. Am J Sports Med 2006;34(5):733–40.
57. Peers K. Extracorporeal shock wave therapy in chronic Achilles and patellar tendinopathy. Leuven, Belgium: Leuven University Press; 2003.
58. Costa ML, Shepsone L, Donell ST, et al. Shock wave therapy for chronic Achilles tendon pain. Clin Orthop Relat Res 2004;440:199–204.
59. Rompe JD. Letter to the editor: shock wave therapy for chronic Achilles tendon pain: a randomized placebo-controlled trial. Clin Orthop Relat Res 2006;445: 276–7.
60. Ohberg L, Alfredson H. Ultrasound guided sclerosis of neovessels in painful chronic Achilles tendinosis: pilot study of a new treatment. Br J Sports Med 2002;36:173–7.
61. Alfredson H, Ohberg L. Sclerosing injections to areas of neo-vascularization reduce pain in chronic Achilles tendinopathy: a double-blind randomized controlled trial. Knee Surg Sports Traumatol Arthrosc 2005;13:338–44.
62. Lind B, Ohberg L, Alfredson H. Sclerosing polidocanol injections in mid-portion Achilles tendinosis: remaining good clinical results and decreased tendon thickness at 2-year follow-up. Knee Surg Sports Traumatol Arthrosc 2006;14: 1327–32.
63. Alfredson H, Ohberg L, Zeisig E. Treatment of midportion Achilles tendinosis: similar clinical results with US and CD-guided surgery outside the tendon and sclerosing polidocanol injections. Knee Surg Sports Traumatol Arthrosc 2007; 15:1504–9.
64. Boesen MI, Torp-Pedersen S, Koenig MJ, et al. Ultrasound guided electrocoagulation in patients with chronic non-insertional Achilles tendinopathy: a pilot study. Br J Sports Med 2006;40:761–6.
65. Fung HL. Clinical pharmacology of organic nitrates. Am J Cardiol 1993;72: 9C–15C.
66. Murrell GAC. Using nitric oxide to treat tendinopathy. Br J Sports Med 2007;41: 227–31.
67. Szomor. Nitric oxide in rotator cuff tendon [PhD thesis]. Sydney: University of New South Wales, 2003.
68. Schaffer MR, Efron PA, Thornton FJ, et al. Nitric oxide, an autocrine regulator of wound fibroblast synthetic function. J Immunol 1997;158:2375–81.

69. Xia W, Szomor Z, Wang Y, et al. Nitric oxide enhances collagen synthesis in cultured human tendon cells. J Orthop Res 2006;24:159–72.
70. Malloy TJ, de Bock C, Wang Y, et al. Gene expression changes in SNAP-stimulated and iNOS-transfected tenocytes: expression of extracellular matrix genes and its implications for tendon healing. J Orthop Res 2006;24:1869–82.
71. Kane TPC, Ismail M, Calder JDF. Topical glyceryl trinitrate and noninsertional Achilles tendinopathy. Am J Sports Med 2008;36(6):1160–3.
72. Murrell GAC, Szabo C, Hannafin JA, et al. Modulation of tendon healing by nitric oxide. Inflamm Res 1997;46:19–27.
73. Szomor ZL, Appleyard RA, Murrell GAC. Overexpression of nitric oxide synthases in tendon overuse. 49th annual Meeting of the Orthopaedic Research Society. New Orleans, LA, February 2–5, 2003;146.
74. Paoloni JA, Appleyard RC, Nelson J, et al. Topical glyceryl trinitrate treatment of chronic noninsertional Achilles tendinopathy. J Bone Joint Surg Am 2004;86(5): 916–22.
75. Paoloni JA, Murrell GAC. Three year followup study of topical glyceryl trinitrate treatment of chronic noninsertional Achilles tendinopathy. Foot Ankle Int 2007; 28(10):1064–8.
76. De Mos M, van El B, DeGroot J, et al. Achilles tendinosis: changes in biomechanical composition and collagen turnover rate. Am J Sports Med 2007;35: 1549–56.
77. Fu S, Chan B, Wang W, et al. Increased expression of matrix metalloproteinase 1 (MMP1) in 11 patients with patellar tendinosis. Acta Orthop Scand 2002;73: 658–62.
78. Ireland D, Harrall R, Curry V, et al. Multiple changes in gene expression in chronic human Achilles tendinopathy. Matrix Biol 2001;20:159–69.
79. Lo I, Marchuk L, Hollinshead R, et al. Matrix metalloproteinase and tissue inhibitor of matrix metalloproteinase mRNA levels are specifically altered in torn rotator cuff tendons. Am J Sports Med 2004;32:1223–9.
80. Capasso G, Mafulli N, Testa V, et al. Preliminary results with peritendinous protease inhibitor injections in the management of Achilles tendinitis. J Sports Traumatol Rel Res 1993;15:37–40.
81. Capasso G, Testa V, Mafulli N, et al. Aprotinin, corticosteroids and normosaline in the management of patellar tendinopathy in athletes: a prospective randomized study. Sports Exerc Injury 1997;3:111–5.
82. Dollery C, editor. Therapeutic drugs. Edinburgh UK: Churchill Livingstone; 1991. p. 73–4.
83. Berton A, Lorimier S, Emonard H, et al. Contribution of the plasmin/matrix metalloproteinase cascade to the retraction of human fibroblast populated collagen lattices. Mol Cell Biol Res Commun 2000;3:173–80.
84. Orchard J, Massey A, Brown R, et al. Successful management of tendinopathy with injections of the MMP-inhibitor aprotinin. Clin Orthop Relat Res 2008;466: 1625–32.
85. Aubin F, Javaudin L, Rochcongar P. Case reports of aprotinin in Achilles tendinopathies with athletes. J Pharmacie Clinique 1997;16:270–3.
86. Komurcu M, Akkus O, Basbozkurt M, et al. Reduction of restrictive adhesions by local aprotinin application and primary sheath repair in surgically traumatized flexor tendons of the rabbit. J Hand Surg Am 1997;22:826–32.
87. Brown R, Orchard J, Kinchington M, et al. Aprotinin in the management of Achilles tendinopathy: a randomized controlled trial. Br J Sports Med 2006;40: 275–9.

88. Rukin NJ, Maffulli N. Systemic allergic reactions to aprotinin injection around the Achilles tendon. J Sci Med Sport 2007;10:320–2.
89. Orchard J, Massey A, Rimmer J, et al. Delay of 6 weeks between aprotinin injections for tendinopathy reduces risk of allergic reaction. J Sci Med Sport 2008;11: 473–80.
90. Stergiolas A, Stergioula M, Aarskog R, et al. Effects of low-level laser therapy and eccentric exercises in the treatment of recreational athletes with chronic Achilles tendinopathy. Am J Sports Med 2008;36(5):881–7.
91. Reddy GK, Stehno-Bittel L, Enwemeka CS. Laser Photostimulation of collagen production in healing rabbit Achilles tendons. Lasers Surg Med 1998;22:281–7.
92. Delbari A, Bayat M, Bayat M. Effect of low-level laser therapy on healing of medial collateral ligament injuries in rats: an ultrastructural study. Photomed Laser Surg 2007;25:191–6.
93. Maxwell NJ, Ryan MB, Taunton JE, et al. Sonographically guided intratendinous injection of hyperosmolar dextrose to treat chronic tendinosis of the Achilles tendon: a pilot study. AJR Am J Roentgenol 2007;189:215–20.
94. Edwards SG, Calandruccio JH. Autologous blood injections for refractory lateral epicondylitis. J Hand Surg 2003;28A:272–8.
95. Connell DA, Ali KE, Ahmad M, et al. Ultrasound-guided autologous blood injection for tennis elbow. Skeletal Radiol 2006;35:371–7.
96. Suresh SP, Ali KE, Jones H, et al. Medial epicondylitis: is ultrasound guided autologous blood injection an effective treatment? Br J Sports Med 2006; 40(11):935–9.
97. James SL, Ali K, Pocock C, et al. Ultrasound guided dry needling and autologous blood injection for patellar tendinosis. Br J Sports Med 2007;41f(8):518–21.
98. Lee TG, Ahmad TS. Intralesional autologous blood injection compared to corticosteroid injection for treatment of chronic plantar fasciitis: a prospective, randomized, controlled trial. Foot Ankle Int 2007;28(9):984–90.
99. Giombini A, Cesare AD, Casciello G, et al. Hyperthermia at 434 MHz in the treatment of overuse sport tendinopathies: a randomized controlled clinical trial. Int J Sports Med 2002;23:207–11.
100. Chapman-Jones D, Hill D. Novel microcurrent treatment is more effective than conventional therapy for chronic Achilles tendinopathy. Physiotherapy 2002; 88:471–9.
101. Sanchez M, Anitua E, Azofra J, et al. Comparison of surgically repaired Achilles tendon tears using platelet-rich fibrin matrices. Am J Sports Med 2007;35(2): 245–51.
102. Virchenko O, Aspenberg P. How can one platelet injection after tendon injury lead to a stronger tendon after 4 weeks? Acta Orthop 2006;77(5):806–12.
103. Bolt P, Clerk AN, Luu HH, et al. BMP-14 gene therapy increases tendon tensile strength in a rat model of Achilles tendon injury. J Bone Joint Surg 2007;89: 1315–20.
104. Majewski M, Betz O, Ochsner PE, et al. Ex vivo adenoviral transfer of BMP-12 cDNA improves Achilles tendon healing in a rat model. Gene Ther 2008;15: 1139–46.

Non-Surgical Management of Achilles Ruptures

Giselle Tan, MD, Brian Sabb, DO, Anish R. Kadakia, MD*

KEYWORDS

- Achilles • Tendon • Rupture • Non-operative • Non-surgical

Incidence of Achilles tendon injuries has increased in recent times as more individuals continue to be active in their later years. The most common scenario is men in their 30s or 40s who play occasional sports (running, basketball, and racquet sports) and increase their training regimen.[1] They commonly recount a sensation of being hit in the back of the calf and may have had calf pain in the past. Although acute rupture of the Achilles tendon is most commonly diagnosed using history and physical examination, improvements in magnetic resonance imaging (MRI) and ultrasonography have led to their routine use in evaluating these injuries and in helping to guide treatment options. Ambrose Pare wrote, "this mischance may be amended by resting in bed but it will never be cured and some relics will remain."[2] The decision to proceed with non-operative or operative management of acute Achilles tendon ruptures has been the subject of much controversy in the current literature, especially in light of non-operative treatment with functional bracing. This article highlights the current controversy and outlines the rationale for non-surgical treatment of acute Achilles tendon ruptures.

Acute Achilles tendon ruptures typically occur 4 to 6 cm proximal to the insertion site of the tendon. Proximal ruptures are reported to be 10% to 15% of all Achilles ruptures and are secondary to degenerative changes. Rupture at the insertion site is rare and has a high association with factors such as a Haglund deformity, history of insertional Achilles tendinosis, and prior steroid therapy in the area. This article focuses on the non-operative treatment of midsubstance tendon ruptures and is not intended to address treatment of insertional Achilles ruptures.

The mechanism for acute rupture of the tendon is typically indirect loading, such as when pushing off with the foot with knee extension as seen in sprinting and jumping sports, or is unexpected dorsiflexion of the ankle with contraction of the calf muscles, such as when stepping into a hole.[3] Direct impact of the tendon (being kicked or hit)

Division of Foot and Ankle Surgery, Department of Orthopedic Surgery, University of Michigan, 2098 South Main Street, Ann Arbor, MI 48103, USA
* Corresponding author.
E-mail address: anishk@med.umich.edu (A.R. Kadakia).

Foot Ankle Clin N Am 14 (2009) 675–684
doi:10.1016/j.fcl.2009.08.004
1083-7515/09/$ – see front matter © 2009 Elsevier Inc. All rights reserved.

leading to rupture is less common and ranges from 1% to 10%. Other causes such as fluoroquinolone treatment, corticosteroid administration, inflammatory arthropathies, metabolic disorders, overpronation of the foot, and poor footwear have all been implicated in acute Achilles tendon rupture.

EPIDEMIOLOGY

The incidence of Achilles tendon ruptures in the general population is unknown but it seems to be increasing. Most ruptures of the Achilles tendon occur during sporting activities.[4] Rupture of the Achilles tendon is more common in men, with a male to female ratio of 1.7:1 to 12:1. The left Achilles tendon is more commonly injured than the right, possibly because most individuals are right-side dominant. Acute ruptures of the Achilles tendon happen typically in men between ages 30 and 40 years, working in white-collar jobs, and playing occasional recreational sports.

DIAGNOSIS/EVALUATION

Patients with acute Achilles tendon ruptures feel as if they have been hit in the calf, have intense pain, and are usually unable to perform a single-limb heel rise. Examination of the extremity with the patient in a prone position and with gentle dorsiflexion from the examiner will usually reveal a palpable gap 2 to 6 cm proximal to the insertion site with a positive result in the Thompson squeeze test.[5] The calf squeeze test, which is credited to Thompson, should be done circumferentially at the thickest portion of the gastrocnemius-soleus complex. An intact tendon will plantarflex the foot in response to the squeeze test as the soleus muscle is deformed, causing the overlying Achilles tendon to bow away from the tibia (**Fig. 1**A, B). In some rare cases, the diagnosis is difficult to establish because plantarflexion strength and a negative result in

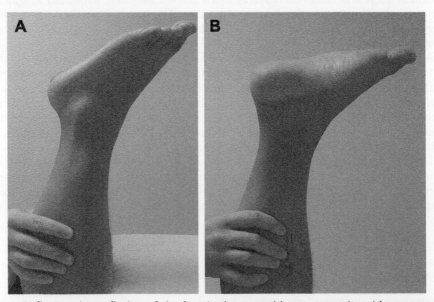

Fig. 1. Reflexive plantarflexion of the foot in the normal lower extremity with squeeze of the calf (*A*). In the injured leg, with squeeze of the calf, there is no significant plantarflexion (*B*). Examining the patient prone and visualizing both extremities facilitates the diagnosis and a discrepancy between the 2 limbs is easily noted.

the squeeze test may be present in an acute rupture if the posterior tibialis, flexor digitorum longus, and flexor hallucis longus muscles are recruited and included in the squeeze test.

Delayed or misdiagnosis of acute Achilles tendon rupture is not uncommon. Inglis and Sculco[6] documented that 23% of acute tendon ruptures were missed by the first doctor to examine the patient. Misdiagnosis may lead to suboptimal treatment, and delay in treating an acute rupture may preclude non-operative management.

IMAGING

Although most acute Achilles tendon ruptures can be clinically diagnosed, tendon evaluation with ultrasonography or MRI allows for an objective and definitive diagnosis and can be helpful in selecting treatment options. Both modalities can be effective in diagnosing full-thickness Achilles tears. Ultrasound evaluation of the Achilles tendon is done with the patient in the prone position with the foot hanging off the bed and in the longitudinal and transverse planes in relation to the tendon itself. The longitudinal sonograms of acute ruptures demonstrate discontinuity of the normal parallel fibrillar pattern, separation of the torn ends, varying amounts of peripheral fluid and echogenic inhomogeneous material in the tendon gap corresponding to hematoma, and adjacent tendinosis. A unique advantage of ultrasonography is the ability to perform dynamic imaging with passive dorsiflexion and plantarflexion, which can be helpful in confirming the full-thickness nature of a tendon tear. In addition, dynamic ultrasonography is the imaging modality of choice[7] to determine if and at what range of motion the tendon ends become apposed. Ultrasound imaging can accurately measure the residual gap of the ruptured tendon ends when non-operative management is being considered (**Fig. 2**).

MRI of Achilles tendon tears is valuable in assessing the gapping of the tendon edges, evaluating partial or interstitial tears, and assessing for fatty degeneration of the soleus muscle to provide an estimate of the chronicity of the tear.[8] The Achilles tendon is usually seen best in the sagittal plane (**Fig. 3**).[9] An acute or partial rupture typically shows a high signal on T2-weighted imaging and the gap distance and the quality of the remnant tendons can be assessed. MRI can also diagnose tennis leg (rupture of the medial head of the gastrocnemius muscle), which responds well to expectant management. Chronic Achilles tendon tears not only demonstrate gapping of the tendon ends but also show continuing atrophy of the soleus muscle, which leads to a decrease in the measured calf circumference and is a predictor of a dysfunctional myotendinous unit.

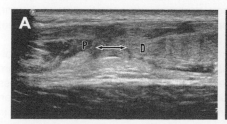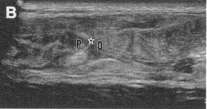

Fig. 2. Full-thickness Achilles tendon tear. (*A*) Longitudinal sonogram with foot in dorsiflexion showing gapping (2-sided arrow) of the tendon ends, confirming a full thickness tear; proximal stump (P) and distal stump (D). (*B*) With passive plantarflexion the torn tendon ends appose (*star*).

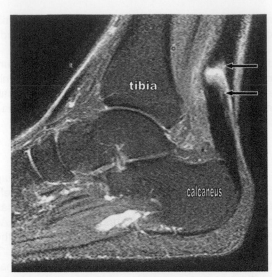

Fig. 3. Full-thickness Achilles tendon tear. Capital T2-weighted fat-saturated MRI shows a tendon gap. The tendon ends are seen (*arrows*) with fluid-filled gap (bright area).

NON-OPERATIVE TREATMENT OF ACUTE RUPTURES

Although operative management predictably results in a good functional outcome and low recurrence of rupture, the adverse outcomes from an anesthetic complication or wound infection can be devastating. These complications are the primary reason behind continued focus on the non-operative management of Achilles ruptures.

The decision to treat an acute Achilles tendon rupture non-operatively relies on several objective measurements using dynamic ultrasound imaging: less than 5 mm of gap with maximum plantarflexion,[10] less than 10 mm of gap with the foot in neutral position, or greater than 75% of tendon apposition with the foot in 20° of plantarflexion.[11,12] The rationale for these criteria is that surgical intervention will result in complete apposition of the tendon remnants; therefore, the requirement must be the same for successful non-operative treatment.[13]

Candidates for non-operative treatment include those with medical comorbidities that preclude an anesthetic or those who cannot tolerate the prone position for surgery. A thorough evaluation for evidence of peripheral vascular disease is important. Systemic disease with thin friable skin or an otherwise unhealthy surgical site may preclude surgery. Smokers and patients with diabetes are at particular risk of wound-edge necrosis. Given the risks of non-operative and operative management, some patients may simply choose non-operative treatment, especially if they meet the criteria mentioned earlier.

Traditional non-operative treatment of acute Achilles tendon ruptures with immobilized casting of the extremity for 8 weeks is no longer justified. There are significant disadvantages such as muscle atrophy, decreased ankle range of motion, and loss of coordination and proprioception. Functional bracing with a refined rehabilitation protocol allows for early motion and improved tendon healing,[14,15] and results in greater patient satisfaction.[16]

The Sheffield splint was the forerunner of functional bracing. Saleh and colleagues[16] randomized 40 patients to conservative management with casting alone for 8 weeks or cast immobilization for 3 weeks followed by controlled early mobilization in a removable 15° plantarflexion ankle-foot orthosis (Sheffield splint). Their results showed improved dorsiflexion motion, decreased time to comfortable ambulation, and improved patient satisfaction with the splint. McComis and colleagues[18] reported on 15 patients who underwent functional bracing in a 45° plantarflexion removable orthosis with a progressive rehabilitation protocol. The protocol limited dorsiflexion and the foot was brought slowly to neutral position over a 5-week period. Ten patients returned to preinjury sports, and 4 patients had a loss of 1 activity level. A cost analysis of functional bracing revealed that the mean cost of operative management was nearly 75% higher than functional bracing.

Wallace and colleagues[19] treated 140 consecutive patients with acute Achilles tendon ruptures non-operatively in 2 stages: (1) with a non–weight-bearing period of 4 weeks in an equinus cast and (2) transition to 4 weeks of weight bearing as tolerated in a removable orthosis in 15° of plantarflexion, with encouragement to perform seated active motion of the ankle and subtalar joints without the orthosis throughout the day. After 4 weeks of use, the orthosis was removed and physical therapy was continued to facilitate return to regular activities. Findings in this study included a 6% rerupture rate and a 98% patient satisfaction rate by questionnaire. In this study, 72% of patients were active in sport. Of these patients: 4% returned to a better activity level, 33% returned to the same level, and 54% to a decreased level. Nine percent were unable to return to activity at a mean of 8 weeks following the removal of the orthosis.

Twaddle and colleagues[20] prospectively randomized 42 patients to receive operative or non-operative treatment and both groups followed the same functional rehabilitation protocol. All patients remained non–weight-bearing with crutches for 6 weeks and were placed in an equinus cast for 10 days. After removal of the cast, all patients were placed in a removable below-knee orthosis with 20° of plantarflexion. All participants were instructed to remove the orthosis for 5 minutes every hour and to perform passive plantarflexion and active ankle dorsiflexion while in the seated position, with emphasis on not dorsiflexing the ankle beyond neutral. After 4 weeks, the orthosis was brought to neutral and the same exercise instructions were reiterated. After 6 weeks, the patients were allowed to bear full weight with the orthosis and at 8 weeks, the orthosis was removed and toe-raising exercises were initiated. Stretching and strengthening exercises were allowed once the patient could initiate toe raising on the injured leg alone. Outcomes measured in both groups included ankle motion in plantarflexion and dorsiflexion, complications, patient satisfaction, and calf circumference from the injured leg compared with the uninjured side. In all outcomes, there was no difference in any of the measured parameters.

Two groups used dynamic ultrasonography to guide their treatment regimen of acute Achilles tendon ruptures. Kotnis and colleagues[10] used an absolute cutoff of 5 mm or more of tendon end gap with the foot in equinus to receive operative management. All other patients received non-operative management. Both groups received the same functional rehabilitation protocol as outlined by Saleh and colleagues.[17] Patients were followed up at 3, 6, and 8 weeks and at 4 and 6 months after injury. Complications in the operative and non-operative group were compared and showed a rerupture rate of 1.5% and 3.4%, respectively. Other complications such as wound infection, chronic pain, deep vein thrombosis, and sural nerve numbness were 7.4% in the operative group and 3.4% in the non-operative group. Calf muscle diameter was decreased by a mean of 1 cm in both groups.

To select patients suitable for the non-operative treatment group, Hufner and colleagues[11] used an absolute cutoff of less than 10 mm of gap with the foot in neutral position and greater than 75% of tendon apposition with the foot in 20° of plantarflexion. Patients were treated with a cast for 1 to 3 days and then placed in the Vario-Stabil high-shaft boot (Orthotech GmBH, Gauting, Germany), which maintains plantarflexion of the foot with a 3-cm hindfoot elevation for a total of 8 weeks. All patients were weight-bearing as tolerated in the boot. Physical therapy with isometric and gait exercises was initiated at 3 weeks. At 4 weeks, the exercises were done without the boot and at 6 weeks, muscle training was increased. The patients were followed up clinically with ultrasound examinations at 4, 8, and 12 weeks. If the ultrasound at 8 weeks revealed a healed tendon, the boot was discontinued and the patient wore insoles with a 1-cm heel rise for 3 months. If the ultrasound did not show healing, the boot was continued for an additional 2 weeks. If rerupture was found, non-operative treatment was prolonged or operative management was performed based on the morphology of the reruptured tendon. Complications and patient satisfaction data were collected. The rerupture rate was 6.4% in 125 patients, 96% were pain free, mean return-to-work time was 4.5 weeks, and 75.2% continued sporting activities at the preinjury level. Calf muscle diameter was decreased by a mean of 2.1 cm compared with the uninjured side.

These studies have demonstrated that functional rehabilitation after an acute Achilles tendon rupture promotes improved range of motion, improved patient satisfaction, and improved calf muscle circumference and that the rate of rerupture is not statistically different to operative management of these injuries. The foot should be kept in 20° of plantarflexion during the initial stages of non-operative treatment, because this increases the blood supply to the overlying skin and decreases the contractility of the plantarflexors during ambulation.[21]

Multiple rehabilitation protocols have resulted in satisfactory outcomes that vary with respect to duration of immobilization and weight bearing. A functional rehabilitation protocol for the non-operative treatment of an Achilles rupture that has been used successfully in the author's practice is outlined in **Table 1**. Patient cooperation is critical to the success of non-operative intervention, and this must be communicated to patients so that they understand their critical role in the treatment protocol.

As with all treatment options, patient selection is of paramount importance. Operative treatment should be considered for high-level athletes, young patients, and those who have chronic ruptures with delayed presentation of 4 or more weeks.[22]

COMPLICATIONS OF NON-OPERATIVE MANAGEMENT OF ACUTE RUPTURES

There have been numerous studies comparing operative and non-operative management of acute Achilles tendon rupture. Cetti and colleagues[4] reported on a prospective study of 111 patients randomly selected to receive operative and non-operative treatment, with physical examination as the means of diagnosing an acute rupture. No imaging studies were reported. After repair or as part of the non-operative treatment regimen, patients were immobilized in short leg casts. Rerupture rates of 5% and 15% were reported in the operative and non-operative groups, respectively. This was not found to be statistically significant. The complication rate in the operative group was 4%, which included deep infection. Return to sport was also followed in both groups, with 57% and 29% return to the same level of sport in the operative and non-operative groups, respectively. Cetti and colleagues[4] also reported on pooled data from review of the literature until 1990. They reported a rerupture rate of 1.4% and 13.4% in the operative and non-operative groups, respectively. Mean plantarflexion strength was found to be 87% in the operative group and 78% in the non-operative group. Although pooled data showed a statistical significance in the rerupture rate between operative and non-operative management, the individual studies did not show any difference between the groups.

Table 1 Protocol for non-operative management of acute Achilles tendon ruptures	
Initial evaluation	Ultrasound or MRI examination showing less than 5 mm of gap with maximum plantarflexion, less than 10 mm, with the foot in neutral position, or greater than 75% of tendon apposition with the foot in 20° of plantarflexion
Initial management	Cast with foot in full equinus with dorsiflexion block; non–weight-bearing
2-week evaluation	Transition to removable cast or cast boot with foot in 20° of plantarflexion with two 1-cm wedges in cast boot; can be WBAT; boot to be worn 24 hours a day
4-week evaluation	Clinical examination: able to palpate continuity of tendon. Recommend repeat ultrasound imaging or MRI to verify that tendon edges are apposed without evidence of gapped ends. If tendon edges not apposed, recommend surgical consideration Boot removed 5 minutes per hour when awake to perform active dorsiflexion to neutral with passive plantarflexion
6-week evaluation	Clinical examination to document continuity of tendon. Removal of one 1-cm wedge. Continue active dorsiflexion to neutral with passive plantarflexion. Initiate physical therapy program to begin proprioception and non-weight-bearing muscle strengthening out of the boot
8-week evaluation	Clinical examination to ensure tendon continuity and evaluation with ultrasonography or MRI to document continued tendon apposition. If lack of tendon healing or continuity, consider operative intervention. If tendon in continuity, recommend transition of boot to daytime wear only without wedge. Continue formal physical therapy program
10-week evaluation	Discontinue use of boot and use a 1-cm heel wedge for 3 more months. May start to ride stationary bike and progress physical therapy program with WBAT in shoe with lift. No sprinting or running until heel wedge is discontinued

Abbreviation: WBAT, weight bearing as tolerated.

In a review of the literature up to 2004, Khan and colleagues[23] found that a pooled rate of rerupture in operative and non-operative treatment of acute Achilles tendon ruptures was 3.5% and 12.6%, respectively. Complications other than rerupture, such as wound infection, adhesions, and sensory deficits, was 34.1% and 2.7% in the operative and non-operative group, respectively. Cast immobilization was also compared with functional bracing and the pooled rerupture rate was 12.2% and 2.4%, respectively. Complications were more common in the cast immobilization group (35.7%), which included adhesions, infection, or keloid formation, than in the functional bracing group (19.5%). The rate of rerupture in the functional bracing group (2.4%) and in the operative treatment group (3.5%) was nearly equivalent.

NON-OPERATIVE MANAGEMENT OF NEGLECTED ACHILLES RUPTURES

Chronically misdiagnosed Achilles tendon ruptures result in significant weakness and altered gait mechanics. Despite the healing response that occurs after a neglected rupture, to repair the defect, the musculotendinous unit is lengthened and therefore cannot shorten sufficiently to generate normal plantarflexion strength. Surgical treatments to reconstruct the Achilles tendon are effective; however, in low-demand or high-risk patients, surgery may not be the most appropriate option. The most common

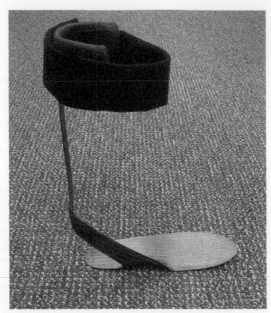

Fig. 4. Carbon fiber AFO. Note the low profile design.

complaints of a patient with a neglected rupture is weakness during toe-off and fatigue with prolonged walking. Patients with neglected ruptures can also complain of heel pain during ambulation, secondary to the dorsiflexed position of the foot during heel strike. Non-operative treatment should address both of these concerns. Use of a rigid ankle-foot orthosis (AFO) can help stabilize the ankle and hindfoot by statically holding the ankle in a neutral position. However, this does not allow dynamic motion of the ankle and therefore does not address the push-off weakness. The rigidity that is created also does not allow for a smooth transition between the stance and swing phases of gait. The use of a rocker bottom shoe can help improve this transition when using a rigid AFO. Solid plastic or rigid AFOs are also bulky and cosmetically displeasing to some patients. Use of a dynamic carbon fiber AFO (**Fig. 4**) that has energy storing capacity helps to reproduce more normal propulsion during toe-off. A carbon fiber AFO is also more lightweight and cosmetically appealing than a typical hard plastic AFO. Although not creating a normal gait for the patient, the dynamic carbon fiber AFO is a simple and effective orthosis for those patients in whom surgical intervention is not warranted.

SUMMARY

1. Acute Achilles tendon tears are becoming more common as individuals stay more active in their later years.
2. An acute tear is typically diagnosed from the patient's history and by examination of the affected foot. Patients typically have a palpable defect, a positive result in the Thompson squeeze test, and are unable to perform a single-limb rise.
3. Ultrasound imaging and MRI can provide accurate diagnosis of an acute Achilles tendon tear and can help evaluate the amount of gap between the tendon edges and the quality of the remnant tendon.

4. Patients showing less than 5 mm of gap between the tendon edges with maximum plantarflexion, 10 mm, with the foot in neutral, or patients showing apposition of the tendon edges with 20° of plantarflexion are candidates for non-operative management.
5. Functional rehabilitation of these patients with a removable cast or boot with minimal restriction of weight bearing and motion leads to increased patient satisfaction and greater likelihood of return to preinjury activities
6. Patients must cooperate with the strict requirements of the non-operative rehabilitation because early discontinuation of immobilization will result in rerupture and a poor outcome.

REFERENCES

1. Jozsa L, Kvist M, Balint BJ, et al. The role of recreational sport activity in Achilles tendon rupture: a clinical, pathoanatomical and sociological study of 292 cases. Am J Sports Med 1989;17:338–43.
2. Klenerman L. The history of the tendo Achillis and its rupture. In: Maffuli N, Almekinders LC, editors. The Achilles tendon. London: Springer; 2007. p.1–4.
3. Arner O, Lindholm A. Subcutaneous rupture of the Achilles tendon: a study of 92 cases. Acta Chir Scand Suppl 1959;239:1–51.
4. Cetti R, Steen-Erik C, Ejsted R, et al. Operative versus non-operative treatment of Achilles tendon rupture: a prospective randomized study and review of the literature. Am J Sports Med 1993;21:791–9.
5. Thompson TC, Doherty JH. Spontaneous rupture of tendon of Achilles. a new clinical diagnostic test. J Trauma 1962;2:126–9.
6. Inglis AE, Sculco TP. Surgical repair of ruptures of the tendo Achillis. Clin Orthop Relat Res 1981;156:160–9.
7. Jacobson JA. Musculoskeletal ultrasound or MRI: which do I choose? Semin Musculoskelet Radiol 2005;9:135–49.
8. Schweitzer ME, Karasick D. MR imaging of disorders of the Achilles tendon. AJR Am J Roentgenol 2000;175:613–25.
9. Helms CA. Fundamentals of skeletal radiology. 3rd edition. Philadelphia: Elsevier Saunders; 2005.
10. Kotnis R, David S, Handley R, et al. Dynamic ultrasound as a selection tool reducing Achilles tendon reruptures. Am J Sports Med 2006;34:1395–400.
11. Hufner TM, Brandes DB, Thermann H, et al. Long-term results after functional non-operative treatment of Achilles tendon rupture. Foot Ankle Int 2006;27:167–71.
12. Poynton AR, O'Rourke K. An analysis of skin perfusion over the Achilles tendon in varying degrees of plantarflexion. Foot Ankle Int 2001;22:572–4.
13. Thermann H, Becher C. Nonoperative management of acute ruptures. In: Nunley JA, editor. The Achilles tendon. New York: Springer; 2009. p. 41–53.
14. Gelberman RH, Woo SL, Lothringer K, et al. Effects of early intermittent passive mobilization on healing canine flexor tendons. J Hand Surg Am 1982;7:170–5.
15. Enwemeka CS, Spielholz NI, Nelson AJ. The effect of early functional activities on experimentally tenotomized Achilles tendons in rats. Am J Phys Med Rehabil 1988;67:264–9.
16. Saleh M, Marshall PD, Senior R, et al. The Sheffield splint for controlled early mobilization after rupture of the calcaneal tendon: a prospective, randomized comparison with plaster treatment. J Bone Joint Surg Br 1992;74:206–9.

17. Gelberman RH, Woo SL, Amiel D, et al. Influences of flexor sheath continuity and early motion on tendon healing in dogs. J Hand Surg Am 1990;15:791–9.
18. McComis GP, Nawoczenski DA, DeHaven KE. Functional bracing for rupture of the Achilles tendon: clinical results and analysis of ground-reaction forces and temporal data. J Bone Joint Surg Am 1997;79:1799–808.
19. Wallace RGH, Traynor IER, Kernohan WG, et al. Combined conservative and orthotic management of acute ruptures of the Achilles tendon. J Bone Joint Surg Am 2004;86:1198–202.
20. Twaddle BC, Poon P. Early motion for Achilles tendon ruptures: is surgery important? A randomized, prospective study. Am J Sports Med 2007;35:2033–8.
21. Akizuki KH, Gartman EJ, Nisonson B, et al. The relative stress on the Achilles tendon during ambulation in an ankle immobiliser: implications for rehabilitation after Achilles tendon repair. Br J Sports Med 2001;35:329–33.
22. Gabel S, Manoli A. Neglected rupture of the Achilles tendon. Foot Ankle Int 1994; 15:512–7.
23. Khan RJK, Fick D, Keogh A, et al. Treatment of acute Achilles tendon ruptures: a meta-analysis of randomized, controlled trials. J Bone Joint Surg Am 2005; 87:2202–10.

Minimal Incision Techniques for Acute Achilles Repair

Mark S. Davies, FRCS (Tr & Orth)[a],*, Matthew Solan, FRCS (Tr & Orth)[a,b,c]

KEYWORDS

- Acute • Rupture • Achilles tendon • Mini-open
- Percutaneous • Repair

Despite hundreds of publications in the medical literature on the subject of acute rupture of the Achilles tendon, the jury remains firmly out as far as agreement is concerned on its optimal treatment. Proponents of nonoperative treatment cite the unacceptably high complication rates of sural nerve damage and wound problems associated with open surgery. Those favoring surgical repair of the acutely ruptured Achilles tendon quote the much higher rerupture rate associated with nonoperative treatment compared with surgical repair as justification for their approach. As with all controversies, there are always two sides to the argument, and this is a subject where controversy is likely to persist for some time yet. In 2005, Movin and colleagues[1] studied 8 review articles published between 1986 and 2004 and found that nonsurgical complication rates ranged from 0% to 10%, whereas the surgical complication rates were as low as 4.7% in one study but as high as 34% in another. However, the rerupture rate associated with nonoperative treatment ranged from 8.4% to 17.7%, whereas in surgical series the rate was as low as 1.4% in one series and less than 3.5% in another.

In 2005, Khan and colleagues[2] conducted a comprehensive meta-analysis of randomized controlled trials pertaining to treatment of acute Achilles tendon ruptures and concluded that open operative treatment of the acutely ruptured Achilles tendon reduced the rerupture rate compared with nonoperative treatment but that operative treatment was associated with a significantly higher risk of other complications. It was

The authors have no financial or professional relationships relevant to the subject matter of this article.

[a] The London Foot and Ankle Centre, The Hospital of St John and St Elizabeth, 60 Grove End Road, London NW8 9NH, UK

[b] Department of Orthopaedic Surgery, Royal Surrey County Hospital, Guildford, Surrey, GU2 7XX, UK

[c] Surrey Foot and Ankle Clinic, Guildford Nuffield Hospital, Stirling Road, Guildford, Surrey, GU2 7RF, UK

* Corresponding author.
E-mail address: markdavies@uk-consultants.co.uk (M.S. Davies).

Foot Ankle Clin N Am 14 (2009) 685–697
doi:10.1016/j.fcl.2009.07.006
1083-7515/09/$ – see front matter © 2009 Elsevier Inc. All rights reserved.

further concluded that percutaneous repairs might be associated with a reduction in overall complication rates and that functional bracing after surgery lowers the overall complication rate.

In the introduction to the December 2007 issue of *Foot and Ankle Clinics of North America*, whose theme was "Tendon Injury and Repair," Myerson[3] wrote, "It would seem that the age-old repeated question of management of an acute rupture of the Achilles tendon has been resolved, and there are very few proponents worldwide who advocate a closed method of treatment." In the same year, Twaddle and Poon[4] published the results of a randomized prospective study on the role of early motion for treatment of acute Achilles tendon ruptures with and without surgical intervention and concluded that there was no significant difference between the two groups; the results included the rerupture rate, which was low in both the operatively treated and the nonoperatively treated groups. They concluded that controlled early motion is the most important aspect of treatment of the acutely ruptured Achilles tendon and not whether the patient was treated surgically or not. The jury remains firmly out!

The aim of this article is therefore not to draw conclusions regarding optimal treatment of the acutely ruptured Achilles tendon but rather to review the subject of minimal incision techniques and the results that can be anticipated from these methods.

THE RATIONALE FOR MINIMAL INCISION SURGERY

If it is accepted that the goal of treatment of the acutely ruptured Achilles is to restore the patient to preinjury levels of activity and to avoid major complications, then the treatment must minimize the risks of infection, sural nerve damage, and rerupture. Any surgeon who has treated enough ruptures of the Achilles tendon has seen the potentially devastating consequences of failed operative and failed nonoperative treatment. **Fig. 1** depicts a 33-year-old man who underwent surgical repair and subsequently developed infection and rerupture of the tendon. **Fig. 2** depicts a 29-year-old man who ruptured his Achilles tendon and was treated nonoperatively with serial casts for 8 weeks; the tendon reruptured spontaneously 3 days after removal of the plaster.

EVOLUTION OF MINIMAL INCISION TECHNIQUES AND THEIR RESULTS

In 1977, Ma and Griffith[5] reported an alternative surgical strategy to address the problems associated with surgical repair. They reported on 18 patients who had been

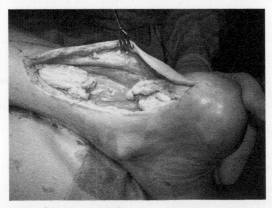

Fig. 1. Infected rerupture after open repair.

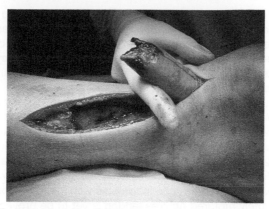

Fig. 2. Rerupture after nonoperative treatment.

treated surgically under local anesthesia and without tourniquet for a closed acute rupture of the Achilles tendon. This is the first report of a percutaneous technique for the treatment of acute closed Achilles tendon ruptures, and the investigators concluded that the preliminary results suggested that this technique was more promising than open repair or short leg equinus casts because it restored tendon length and strength and at the same time minimized postoperative complications. This was not a randomized trial, and there were only 18 patients in the study. However, it showed that effective restoration of tendon function could be achieved surgically without an open approach. Although Ma and Griffith had no problems with iatrogenic injury to the sural nerve, Klein and colleagues[6] reported an alarming 13% incidence of sural nerve damage associated with the technique of Ma and Griffith.

Because the sural nerve is vulnerable to iatrogenic injury during percutaneous repair of the Achilles, its course has been described and redescribed in many papers and textbooks. One would imagine that the course of the nerve has not changed much over the centuries, but its course has nevertheless been the subject of much study. There is no doubt that the position of the sural nerve is variable and therefore there is no rigid anatomic landmark that can be used to avoid damage to it by a "blindly" placed suture needle. Webb and colleagues[7] published the results of dissection of the sural nerve in 30 cadaveric specimens and declared that at the level of the Achilles tendon insertion into the calcaneum, the sural nerve was a mean 18.8 mm anterior and lateral from the lateral border of the tendon. More proximally, and in keeping with other studies, the sural nerve crosses the lateral border of the Achilles tendon approximately 9.8 cm from the calcaneum. They therefore concluded that percutaneous sutures should not be placed in the lateral half of the Achilles tendon. On the basis of this conclusion, Webb and Bannister[8] described a new technique of minimal incision surgery to avoid damage to the sural nerve. This technique involved making three midline stab incisions over the posterior aspect of the tendon. Using a no. 1 nylon suture on a 90-mm cutting needle, the tendon ends are approximated with two box stitches. They reviewed 27 patients who had undergone this technique, and the median interval from surgery was almost 3 years. There was one case of mild wound problem and one case of complex regional pain syndrome, but there were no cases of rerupture or sural nerve injury. In 1995, Wagnon and Akayi[9] conducted a subsequent retrospective study of the Webb-Bannister technique on 57 patients. They compared the technique to a conventional open repair and found similar functional results but a lower complication rate associated with the minimal incision technique.

The sural nerve remains at risk with minimal incision surgery, and there are strategies other than placement of midline stab incisions to avoid damage to it. In 2006, Majewski and colleagues[10] published an article on the subject of avoiding sural nerve damage during percutaneous repair of the Achilles tendon. They retrospectively studied 84 patients treated at two different hospitals where a similar minimal incision surgical technique was used to repair acutely ruptured Achilles tendons. In one hospital, however, the technique involved an additional minimal incision to expose and therefore to protect the sural nerve before suture placement. In the group in which the sural nerve was not exposed, there was an 18% incidence of sural nerve–related complications, whereas there were no such problems in the group in which the nerve was exposed. In 2007, Flavin and colleagues[11] described a clinical test to map the sural nerve and found a good correlation with simultaneous ultrasonic mapping. This study was performed, however, in individuals with intact tendons, and the value of its use in the acutely ruptured Achilles tendon is yet to be proven.

In the authors' institution it is a routine practice to examine with ultrasound the acutely ruptured Achilles tendon. This allows confirmation of the diagnosis, accurate marking of the tendon ends, and assessment of whether the tendon ends come together on passive plantar flexion. At the same time, it allows the precise location of the sural nerve as it crosses the Achilles tendon, thereby minimizing further risk of sural nerve damage.

With the perception that minimal incision surgery had advantages over open repair and nonoperative repairs, modification and new innovative techniques were bound to follow. In 2002, Assal and colleagues[12] published the results of a prospective multi-center study using a limited open repair and a specially designed instrument (**Fig. 3**; Achillon device, Integra LifeSciences Corporation, Plainsboro, NJ, USA) to ensure that all the sutures were placed within the paratenon, therefore minimizing the risk of placing suture material within the sural nerve. It does not eliminate the risk of needle damage to the sural nerve, but in their series there were no cases of sural nerve impairment postoperatively. This is the technique preferred by the authors and is described in more detail in the following sections.

Other methods include the techniques described by Delponte and colleagues[13] in 1992, Gorschewsky and colleagues[14] in 2004, and Amlang and colleagues[15] in 2006. Delponte and colleagues devised a modified percutaneous technique using a harpoon device known as the "Tenolig" device (Fournitures Hospitalieres Industrie,

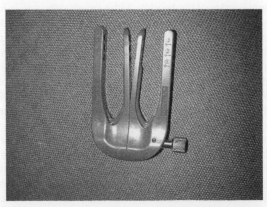

Fig. 3. Achillon device.

Quimper, France). In this procedure, two small incisions are made approximately 5 cm proximal to the ruptured tendon. The harpoon is passed down through the rupture site, either side of the Achilles insertion in the os calcis, and is secured proximally with barbs and distally using lead crimps, having tensioned the tendon at the correct length. The device is removed at 6 weeks postsurgery. Although the device is capable of restoring tendon length and continuity "percutaneously," it has been associated with unacceptably high complication rates, as exemplified by Maes and colleagues[16] in 2006. The disadvantages of the device are that the device is inside the tendon but it is secured externally and that it needs to be removed at 6 weeks, which is an early stage in the healing process, thus leaving no support for the healing tendon. Maes and colleagues[16] described the outcome of Achilles tendon repair in 124 cases (79 men and 45 women, with an average age of 41.5 years) using the harpoon device. They encountered five cases of unbending of the wire, one case of rupture of the wire, and 12 cases of tendon rerupture. There were ten cases of skin necrosis at the entry point of the device and eight sural nerve injuries. Their conclusion was that they preferred a limited open approach, which allows visualization of the tendon ends and confirmation of tendon end apposition. Gorschewsky and colleagues[14] reported the results of a modification of the harpoon technique and the usage of a fibrin sealant through a small incision at the rupture site, which was identified preoperatively by ultrasound. Their results of 64 patients were more favorable than those of Maes and colleagues, with no sural nerve problems and all patients returning to sport at an average duration of five and a half months after surgery.

In 2006, Amlang and colleagues[15] described their results using the Dresden instrument in 61 patients (62 cases). This technique involves a proximal incision and then insertion of the instrument, which places the suture in the interval between the lower leg fascia and the peritenon with the threads running in a "paratendinous" direction. There were two (3.2%) cases of rerupture and no cases of sural nerve injury. There was also one case of late superficial infection. The investigators quoted a 62% "very good" and a 30% "good" result rate with an average American Orthopaedic Foot and Ankle Society (AOFAS) score of 96 points (78–100 points). Despite these encouraging results, neither the Dresden instrument nor the harpoon tenorrhaphy technique has become popular in the United Kingdom to date.

Apart from sural nerve issues, one of the major drawbacks associated with the percutaneous method of repair is the failure to appose the tendon ends and/or creation of malalignment of the tendon ends as a consequence of not visualizing the tendon ends. Another drawback is the lower strength of the repair that is achieved using minimally invasive techniques. Hockenbury and Johns[17] showed in cadaveric specimens that openly repaired tendons were able to tolerate twice the degree of ankle dorsiflexion before a 10-mm gap appeared when compared with those repaired using Ma and Griffith's technique. To a certain extent, this finding is not particularly relevant to the clinical situation with acutely ruptured tendons in living humans, because postoperative rehabilitation programs do not involve forcing the ankle into dorsiflexion in the early postoperative period. However, modifications of Ma and Griffith's technique, devised by Cretnik and colleagues,[18] using more suture passes, have overcome the problem with tendon gapping on load testing. In addition, a later study by Cretnik and colleagues[19] showed an equivalent functional outcome using their technique when compared with an open technique that had a lower overall complication rate, but there were still cases of sural nerve disturbance and rerupture in both groups.

The argument for limited open/percutaneous repair of the acutely ruptured Achilles tendon was further strengthened in 1995 with the publication of Kakiuchi's[20] series, in which his repair method in 12 patients was compared with ten open repairs. Although the series was small and no scoring system was used, the two groups were assessed using subjective and objective measures, and the results were significantly better in the limited open/percutaneous group. These results are backed up by the retrospective study of Rebeccato and colleagues,[21] in which 52 patients were assessed after open, percutaneous, or mini-open plus percutaneous repair. The outcome measures were strength, performance, time of return to work, range of motion, and calf circumference, and the best results were achieved using the technique of Kakiuchi.

The evolution of surgical repair of the Achilles tendon has been described earlier, and it would seem that to achieve the desired outcome of return to preinjury levels of activity and to incur as low a complication rate as possible, the best procedure is one without an open approach but with a percutaneous method that allows accurate apposition of the tendon ends without interposed tissue. This necessitates a mini-open approach at the rupture site with preoperative mapping of the sural nerve, with the visualization of the sural nerve at surgery, or with a suture technique, which categorically avoids the nerve. In addition, the repair needs to be as robust as that achieved with an open repair. The authors believe that the Achillon device, devised by Assal and colleagues,[12] provides the best method to achieve the previously stated goals of return to preinjury levels of activity while minimizing the complication rate.

Assal and colleagues developed the Achillon device based on the principles of Kakiuchi's mini-open/percutaneous technique and subsequently published their results after using the device in 82 patients, although they excluded three patients with early reruptures, one of whom had fallen off a bicycle and the other two being noncompliant. A mean AOFAS score of 96 points was achieved when the patients were followed up at an average of 26 months postoperation. Isokinetic and endurance testing showed no significant differences between the injured and uninjured sides. In addition, there were no wound problems or sural nerve issues, and the only reruptures were those that were excluded from the study. Calder and Saxby[22] (Brisbane, Australia), subsequently published the outcome in 46 patients after using the Achillon device, which they used through a horizontal incision rather than a longitudinal incision. There were no cases of rerupture, two cases of temporary sural nerve paresthesia, and one case of superficial wound infection. An average AOFAS score of 98.4 points (range, 95–100 points) was obtained, and all the patients returned to previous levels of sporting activity by 6 months. Ismail and colleagues[23] have tested the strength of the repair using the Achillon device in sheep's Achilles tendons and found that the tensile strength was comparable to that achieved with a two-strand Kessler technique, thus giving further evidence that the Achillon device is suitable for repair of the acutely ruptured Achilles tendon.

One of the authors (MSD) has used the Achillon device for all acute ruptures of the Achilles tendon (treated surgically) for the past 6 years. The longest interval between rupture and surgery was 21 days. In one case of a "sleeve" type rupture, it was not possible to effect a repair with the device, and the wound was extended proximally and distally to allow an anatomic repair. The device was used for ruptures of the Achilles tendon, irrespective of the location (ie, including musculotendinous junction ruptures), except those within 4 cm of the insertion to the os calcis. In more than 60 cases, there was one early wound problem,not related to infection but to a bulky suture knot (1 polydioxanone), which penetrated the skin and necessitated its removal 4 weeks post surgery. There have been no wound infections and no sural nerve problems, but it is worth noting, from Atinga and colleagues[24] case report of sural nerve damage using the Achillon device, that careful insertion of the device

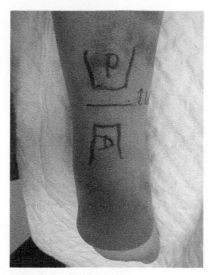

Fig. 4. Skin markings. P, proximal; D, distal.

at the time of surgery is essential, particularly when addressing the proximal tendon stump. In their case, a breach of the paratenon led to inadvertent sural nerve entrapment with suture material. In the authors' series, as in the study of Assal and colleagues, the cases of rerupture and partial rerupture were related to patient noncompliance. One 82-year-old patient at 7 weeks postsurgery was not wearing his brace when he dropped something, and when he attempted to catch it, he sustained a rerupture, which was treated conservatively. Two patients fell while on crutches and felt tearing sensations. Subsequent ultrasound scanning revealed tendon end retraction but intact sutures. Plantar flexion resulted in reapposition of

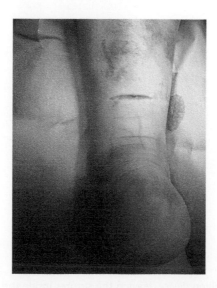

Fig. 5. Skin incision.

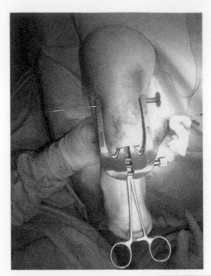

Fig. 6. Achillon device in proximal stump.

the tendon ends as shown on ultrasound, and therefore these partial reruptures were treated with a 2-week period of plaster immobilization in full equinus before resuming the rehabilitation program. One patient sustained a similar partial rerupture with tendon end retraction without suture rupture while participating in sexual activity without his protective brace, and he was treated in a similar manner. A woman had excessive lengthening of the tendon during the postoperative period despite a sound repair at the time of tendon rupture and compliance with the postoperative rehabilitation program. At the 12-month mark, she had unacceptable calf atrophy and weakness necessitating Achilles tendon shortening.

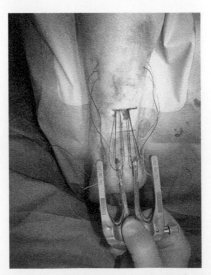

Fig. 7. Removing the Achillon device, leaving the sutures inside the paratenon.

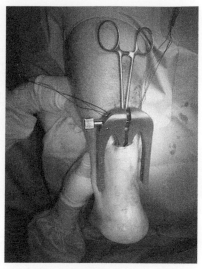

Fig. 8. Achillon device in distal stump.

ACHILLON TECHNIQUE

The procedure is performed with the patient prone, and although the procedure can be performed under local anesthesia without a tourniquet, the authors prefer general anesthesia and the usage of a tourniquet with one dose of prophylactic antibiotics. The tendon ends are marked pre- or peroperatively (**Fig. 4**), and a 3-cm transverse incision is made 1 cm distal to the proximal stump (**Fig. 5**). The paratenon is incised transversely under direct vision, and care is needed particularly with the high ruptures to avoid iatrogenic injury to the sural nerve. A plane is then developed to allow insertion of the Achillon device. The proximal tendon end is held with a clip while the device is inserted within the paratenon (**Fig. 6**). Three absorbable sutures (1 gauge) of different colors and material are then passed through the holes in the device. On withdrawal of the device, the inner arm ensures that the sutures are through the tendon and within the paratenon (**Fig. 7**). This maneuver is repeated for the distal stump (**Fig. 8**). Using

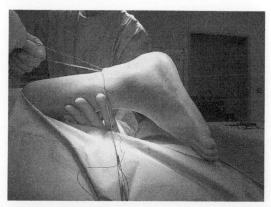

Fig. 9. Sutures in situ distally, with no tension.

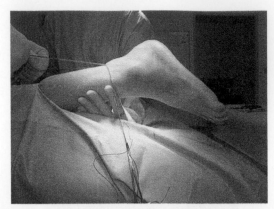

Fig. 10. Tension shows sutures to be in the tendon.

three different colored sutures allows easy identification of the correct suture ends. After insertion of the sutures into the distal stump, it is easy to verify whether the sutures are correctly located by gently pulling on the sutures (**Figs. 9** and **10**). The three sutures on one side are tied first, and then the three on the other side are tied under tension with the ankle fully plantar flexed (**Fig. 11**). With the appropriate tying technique, the suture ends disappear into the repair site and are, therefore, unlikely to penetrate the skin. The paratenon is closed with an absorbable suture, and the skin is closed with two 3-0 nylon sutures. Local anesthetic is infiltrated and the wound dressed, and a below-knee back slab is applied in full equinus. The patient mobilizes non–weight bearing on crutches, and the sutures are removed at 2 weeks. Thrombo-prophylaxis is administered for the first 2 weeks. At 2 weeks, a removable hinged brace is applied and the rehabilitation program commenced. The authors have developed a rehabilitation protocol from studies that have confirmed the beneficial effect of early mobilization after Achilles tendon repair. The authors' rehabilitation protocol is outlined in Appendix 1.

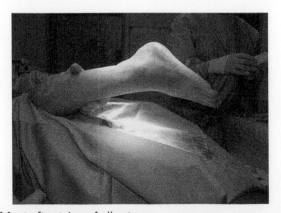

Fig. 11. Position of foot after tying of all sutures.

SUMMARY

Lack of robust prospective randomized studies on the treatment of Achilles tendon rupture makes it impossible to draw conclusions on optimal treatment strategies. The bulk of the evidence available suggests that surgical repair reduces rerupture rates compared with nonoperatively treated tendon ruptures. Surgery does have potential complications, but as outlined in the article, using a mini-open/percutaneous technique of repair might result in highly satisfactory outcomes with acceptably low complication rates. An ideal treatment that results in rapid restoration of normal function without the risk of complication does not exist at the moment.

REFERENCES

1. Movin T, Ryberg A, McBride D, et al. Acute rupture of the Achilles tendon. Foot Ankle Clin 2005;10(2):331–56.
2. Khan R, Fick D, Keogh A, et al. Treatment of acute Achilles tendon ruptures. A meta-analysis of randomized, controlled trials. J Bone Joint Surg Am 2005;87: 2202–10.
3. Myerson M. Foreword. Foot Ankle Clin North Am 2007;12(4):ix–x.
4. Twaddle B, Poon P. Early motion for Achilles tendon ruptures: is surgery important? A randomized, prospective study. Am J Sports Med 2007;35:2033–8.
5. Ma G, Griffith T. Percutaneous repair of acute closed ruptured Achilles tendon: a new technique. Clin Orthop Relat Res 1977;128:247–55.
6. Kloin W, Lang DM, Saleh M. The use of the Ma Griffith technique for percutaneous repair of fresh ruptured tendo Achillis. Chir Organi Mov 1991;76(3):223–8.
7. Webb J, Moorjani J, Radford M. Anatomy of the sural nerve and its relation to the Achilles tendon. Foot Ankle Int 2000;21(6):475–7.
8. Webb JM, Bannister GC. Percutaneous repair of the ruptured tendo Achillis. J Bone Joint Surg Br 1999;81(5):877–80.
9. Wagnon R, Akayi M. The Webb-Bannister percutaneous technique for acute Achilles' tendon ruptures: a functional and MRI assessment. J Foot Ankle Surg 2005;44(6):437–44.
10. Majewski M, Rohrbach M, Czaja S, et al. Avoiding sural nerve injuries during percutaneous Achilles tendon repair. Am J Sports Med 2006;34(5):793–8.
11. Flavin R, Gibney RG, O'Rourke SK. A clinical test to avoid sural nerve injuries in percutaneous Achilles tendon repairs. Injury 2007;38(7):845–7.
12. Assal M, Jung M, Stern R, et al. Limited open repair of Achilles tendon ruptures: a technique with a new instrument and findings of a prospective multicenter study. J Bone Joint Surg Am 2002;84(2):161–70.
13. Delponte P, Potier L, de Poulpiquet P, et al. Treatment of subcutaneous ruptures of the Achilles tendon by percutaneous tenorraphy. Rev Chir Orthop Reparatrice Appar Mot 1992;78(6):404–7 [in French].
14. Gorschewsky O, Pitzl M, Putz A, et al. Percutaneous repair of the Achilles tendon. Foot Ankle Int 2004;25(4):219–24.
15. Amlang M, Christiani P, Heinz P, et al. The percutaneous suture of the Achilles tendon with the Dresden instrument. Oper Orthop Traumatol 2006;18(4): 287–99.
16. Maes R, Copin G, Averous C. Is percutaneous repair of the Achilles tendon a safe technique? A study of 124 cases. Acta Orthop Belg 2006;72(2):179–83.
17. Hockenbury R, Johns J. A biomechanical in vitro comparison of open versus percutaneous repair of tendon Achilles. Foot Ankle 1990;11(2):67–72.

18. Cretnik A, Zlapipah L, Smrkolj V. The strength of percutaneous methods of repair of the Achilles tendon: a biomechanical study. Med Sci Sports Exerc 2000;32(1): 16–20.
19. Cretnik A, Kasanovic M, Smorkolj V. Percutaneous versus open repair of the ruptured Achilles tendon: a comparative study. Am J Sports Med 2005;33(9): 1369–79.
20. Kakiuchi M. A combined open and percutaneous technique for repair of tendo Achillis: comparison with open repair. J Bone Joint Surg Br 1995;77(1):60–3.
21. Rebeccato A, Santini S, Salmaso G, et al. Repair of the Achilles tendon rupture: a functional comparison of three surgical techniques. J Foot Ankle Surg 2001; 40(4):188–94.
22. Calder J, Saxby T. Independent evaluation of a recently described Achilles tendon repair technique. Foot Ankle Int 2006;27(2):93–6.
23. Ismail M, Karim A, Shulman R, et al. The Achillon Achilles tendon repair: is it strong enough? Foot Ankle Int 2008;29(8):808–13.
24. Atinga M, Highland A, Davies MB. The anatomy of the fascia cruris and implications for Achillon limited open Achilles tendon repair: a case report. Foot Ankle Int 2008;29(8):814–6.

APPENDIX 1: REHABILITATION PROTOCOL

Postrepair of ruptured Achilles tendon (Achillon device)
Weeks 1 to 2
- Immobilize in plaster of paris (POP) back slab set in plantar flexion as determined by surgeon at the time of surgery
- Stay in POP full time
- Mobilize non–weight bearing on crutches
- No ankle movement
- Routine care of adjacent joints and other care aspects taught to patient before discharge from hospital

Weeks 2 to 4
- Out of POP and DonJoy (Vista, CA, USA) fixed ankle brace fitted in plantar flexion
- Continue to mobilize non–weight bearing on crutches
- Patient to stay in brace at home at all times, including during sleep
- Supervised exercises only
- No unsupervised exercise. Outpatient physiotherapy to include
- Muscle stimulation 2 times per week
- Active assisted plantar flexion, dorsiflexion, inversion, eversion
- Swelling control
- Soft tissue work and scar mobilization
- Gentle passive non–weight bearing calf stretches
- Brace adjustment to bring ankle toward plantar grade in line with dorsiflexion range is achieved in each treatment session. Allow movement between plantar flexion and dorsiflexion barrier, rather than fixing brace at one angle

Weeks 4 to 6
- Unsupervised range of motion (ROM) exercise permitted
- Progress ROM exercises, active in all directions. Can add Thera-Band (Akron, OH, USA) resistance at week 5
- Continue soft tissue work
- Can use exercise bike
- Aim for neutral dorsiflexion by week 6

- Commence partial weight bearing in brace with crutches at week 4, increasing amount of weight bearing between weeks 4 and 6

Weeks 6 to 8

- Can progress to full weight bearing (FWB) in brace without aid starting from week 6
- Commence weight bearing calf stretches at week 6
- Commence double leg heel raises
- Aim for FWB independently by week 8

Weeks 8 to 12

- Remove brace at week 8 if functional dorsiflexion has been achieved. Use heel lifts in shoes or shoes with a small heel until week 12
- Graded increase of weight bearing activity
- Continue lengthening and strengthening work, exercise bike, gait re-education
- Proprioceptive training

Weeks 12+

- Begin single leg heel raises or progress from 50/50 double heel raises to increased load on affected side
- Start jogging on trampoline and use treadmill via a walk-run program
- Eventually progress to 20-min outdoor running before adding, cutting, and figure-8 drills
- Plyometrics, for example, double to single jumps/hops/lunges on toes, and acceleration or deceleration work
- Sport-specific exercises as required

Open Repair of Acute Achilles Tendon Ruptures

Seth Rosenzweig, MD[a], Frederick M. Azar, MD[b],*

KEYWORDS

- Achilles tendon • Acute rupture • Open repair
- Techniques • Outcomes

Although the Achilles tendon is the strongest in the body, it also is the most often ruptured. Achilles tendon rupture most often occurs during sports activities in middle-aged men. The most frequent mechanism of injury is forced eccentric loading of a planar flexed foot, but ruptures of the Achilles tendon also may occur as the result of direct trauma or as the end result of Achilles paratenonitis, with or without tendinosis. Most Achilles tendon tears occur in the substance of the tendon, approximately 2 to 6 cm above the calcaneal insertion.[1–4]

Risk factors associated with Achilles tendon rupture include:[5]

- Recreational athlete ("weekend warrior")
- Relatively older age (30 to 50 years)
- Previous Achilles tendon injury or rupture
- Previous tendon injections or fluoroquinolone use
- Abrupt changes in training, intensity, or activity level
- Participation in a new activity

Reports of the treatment of Achilles tendon ruptures date back to 1575, when Ambroise Paré[6] described the use of taping and casts, which resulted in suboptimal outcomes. Despite the frequency of the injury and the long history of its treatment, the indications for and superiority of nonoperative or operative management of Achilles tendon rupture remain controversial. In the early twentieth century, closed treatment was widely accepted as the standard of care, but with the increasing functional demands of the athletic population and improved surgical techniques, operative treatment has become a more popular treatment method. Several investigators have reported rerupture rates ranging from 10% to 20% in conservatively managed

[a] Dauterive Orthopaedics and Sports Medicine, 500 North Lewis Street, Suite 280, New Iberia, LA 70563, USA
[b] Department of Orthopaedic Surgery, Campbell Clinic, University of Tennessee, 1211 Union Avenue, Suite 510, Memphis, TN 38104, USA
* Corresponding author.
E-mail address: fazar@campbellclinic.com (F.M. Azar).

Foot Ankle Clin N Am 14 (2009) 699–709
doi:10.1016/j.fcl.2009.07.002
1083-7515/09/$ – see front matter © 2009 Elsevier Inc. All rights reserved.

patients, and higher rates of wound complications in surgically treated patients (2%–20%).[7–18] Rettig and colleagues, in a series of 89 open repairs, found a rerupture rate of 4% and a wound complication rate approaching 4%, leading them to advocate surgical repair of Achilles ruptures.[19]

Few studies have directly compared the outcomes of operative and nonoperative treatment. In a level I prospective study of 111 patients with acute ruptures, Cetti and colleagues found a higher rate of rerupture in those treated nonoperatively (13%) than in those treated operatively (4%,) and a lower return to previous sports or activity (29% compared with 58%). Two deep infections occurred in the operative group.[16] Wong and colleagues, in a quantitative review of operative and nonoperative management of Achilles tendon ruptures, identified 125 articles reporting outcomes of 5370 patients, including 645 treated nonoperatively and 4001 who had open repair.[20] Rerupture rates were 11% in those treated nonoperatively, compared with 2.2% in those treated with open repair and immobilization and 1.4% in those treated with open repair and early mobilization. Skin-healing complications were lowest in those treated nonoperatively (0.5%) and highest in those treated with open repair and immobilization (14.6%). General complication rates were lowest in those treated with open repair and early mobilization (6.7%). Inglis and colleagues compared strength, power, and endurance in 48 patients treated operatively and 31 patients treated nonoperatively, and found all to be significantly greater in the operative group.[21]

Operative repair of acute Achilles tendon ruptures is indicated in active and athletic individuals who wish to resume their activities at their preinjury levels. Age alone should not be considered a contraindication, because good results can be obtained in older patients, many of whom have active lifestyles that involve sports participation. Rettig and colleagues found a rerupture rate of 16.6% in 24 patients younger than 30 years compared with no reruptures in 65 patients older than 30 years after open repair and early mobilization.[19] Contraindications to operative repair include arterial insufficiency, poor skin and soft tissue quality, poorly controlled medical comorbidities (such as diabetes), and inability to comply with an appropriate postoperative rehabilitation protocol.

Operative repair of a ruptured Achilles tendon can be accomplished with a variety of techniques ranging from open repair, to minimally invasive technique, to endoscopic-assisted repair. Each has its proponents and detractors, and the choice of procedure must be individualized based on the patient's age, rehabilitation potential, and activity expectations, as well as the preferences and experience of the surgeon.

OPEN REPAIR OF ACHILLES TENDON RUPTURES

For repair of an acute (<4 weeks) Achilles rupture, several suture techniques, suture materials, and graft materials have been described, including

- End-to-end repair (Bunnell, Krackow, pullout wire)[17,18,21–24]
- End-to-end repair with plantaris reinforcement[25,26]
- Fascial flaps[21,27,28]
- Synthetic grafts[26,29,30]
- Direct repair with allograft augmentation[25]

GENERAL OPERATIVE CONSIDERATIONS

The goal of surgical treatment is to restore the anatomic length of the triceps surae by approximating the ruptured tendon ends. The repair of the Achilles can be done with general[21,25,28] or regional/local anesthesia.[23,31–33] The optimal time to repair without compromising functional results is within the first 30 days of rupture. Preoperative soft tissue normalization is paramount in preventing postoperative complications.[34–36] In a series by Bruggerman and colleagues, patients with the risk factors diabetes, tobacco use, and steroid use had a 42% complication rate following surgical repair compared with a 6% complication rate without these factors.[36]

SURGICAL TECHNIQUES
Open End-to-End Repair

The patient is placed prone with a thigh tourniquet for hemostasis. The contralateral extremity also can be draped for comparison of resting length. A 6- to 8-cm longitudinal incision typically follows the medial edge of the Achilles tendon, but laterally and centrally based incisions have been advocated.[37–39] Medial placement avoids the sural nerve, allows the plantaris to be accessed easily, and minimizes postoperative skin breakdown.[40] The subcutaneous tissue and fat are divided until the crural fascia overlying the tendon is reached. Care must be taken not to undermine the skin. The ankle is plantar flexed to expose and approximate the tendon ends. The tendon ends can be left alone and approximated without debridement. In biomechanical studies, the Krackow technique has proven stronger than either the Bunnell or Kessler suture configuration,[41] but this has not been proven to have clinical significance. Newer polyester sutures have significantly higher failure strength than traditional polyester material. The paratenon may have to be divided further to expose the tendon ends. The final repair is reinforced with interrupted sutures. The foot position should match the contralateral side (resting equinus). Excessive debridement may cause overtightening and prompt the need for advancement. Closure of the paratenon layer following tendon repair reduces skin tension and prevents adhesions. Biomechanical testing also demonstrates that this paratenon closure significantly increases the strength of the final repair.[42] The skin is then closed with an interrupted 3-0 nylon monofilament closure.

Open End-to-End Repair (Mandelbaum)

With the patient prone, a posteromedial incision approximately 10 cm long is made about 1 cm medial to the tendon, ending proximal to where the shoe counter strikes the heel. The skin, subcutaneous tissues, and tendon sheath are sharply dissected. Reflecting the tendon sheath with the subcutaneous tissue minimizes subcutaneous dissection. The ruptured ends of the tendon are approximated with a #2 nonabsorbable suture using a Krackow suture configuration (**Fig. 1**). Keeping the sutures anterior will help decrease the bulk against the skin once the knots are tied. Four strands are biomechanically stronger than 2 strands,[43–45] but often cannot fit onto the tendon. The stability of the repair is checked after the sutures are tied, and the paratenon and subcutaneous tissues are closed with 4-0 absorbable sutures. After skin closure, a sterile dressing and a posterior splint or short leg cast with the foot in gravity equinus are applied.

End-to-End Repair with Plantaris Reinforcement (Lynne)

If the repair is done with the first 2 weeks after rupture, the plantaris tendon can be used to reinforce an end-to-end repair (**Fig. 2**). After this period of time, it scars into the defect of the rupture. After end-to-end repair as described earlier, the plantaris is removed from its insertion onto the calcaneus, fanned out into a membrane, and laid on top of the repair. If possible, the repair should be covered for 1 inch (2.5 cm) on each side of the rupture. Multiple interrupted 2-0 absorbable sutures can be used to tack the plantaris down to the Achilles tendon.

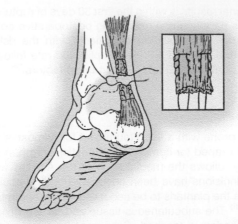

Fig.1. Krackow suture technique for Achilles tendon repair. (*From* Mandelbaum BR, Myerson MS, Forster R. Achilles tendon ruptures: a new method of repair, early range of motion, and functional rehabilitation. Am J Sports Med 1995;23:392–5; with permission.)

Fascial Turn-Down Augmentation (Lindholm)

Another method of repairing ruptures of the Achilles tendon reinforces the sutures with living fascia and prevents adhesion of the repaired tendon to the overlying skin. Two flaps are fashioned from the proximal tendon and gastrocnemius aponeurosis, each approximately 1 cm wide and 7 to 8 cm long (**Fig. 3**). These flaps are left attached at a point 3 cm proximal to the site of rupture. Each flap is turned 180° on itself so that its smooth external surface lies next to the subcutaneous tissue as it is turned distally over the rupture. Each flap is sutured to the distal stump of the tendon and

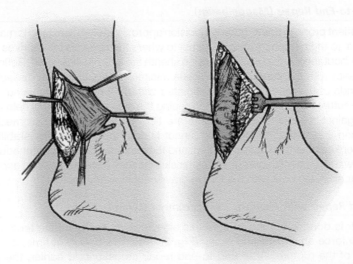

Fig. 2. Plantaris tendon reinforcement of Achilles tendon repair. (*From* Lynn TA. Repair of the torn Achilles tendon, using the plantaris tendon as a reinforcing membrane. J Bone Joint Surg Am 1966;48:268–2; with permission.)

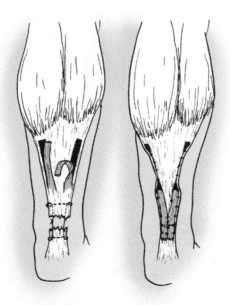

Fig. 3. Achilles tendon repair with fascial reinforcement. (*From* Lindholm A. A new method of operation in subcutaneous rupture of the Achilles tendon. Acta Chir Scand 1959;117: 261–70; with permission.)

to one another so that they cover the site of rupture completely. The wound is closed with care to approximate the tendon sheath over the site of repair.

As a modification of this technique, a single strip of gastrocnemius fascia, approximately 4 cm wide, can be rotated on its distal pedicle and turned distally to cover the rupture site.

Peroneus Brevis Weave Technique (Turco)

The Achilles tendon and the tuberosity of the calcaneus are exposed through a posterolateral longitudinal incision. The sural nerve is identified in the proximal part of the wound and retracted. The peroneus brevis tendon is detached from its insertion through a small incision at the base of the fifth metatarsal. The aponeurotic septum is excised, separating the lateral and posterior compartments, and the freed peroneus brevis is delivered into the first incision. The tuberosity of the calcaneus is dissected, and a hole large enough for passage of the tendon is drilled through the transverse diameter of the bone. The peroneus brevis tendon is passed through this hole and back proximally beside the Achilles tendon, reinforcing the site of rupture, and sutured to the peroneus brevis itself, producing a dynamic loop (**Fig. 4**).

Turco and Spinella described a modification of this technique in which the peroneus brevis is passed through a midcoronal slit in the distal stump of the Achilles tendon. The graft is sutured medially and laterally to the stump and proximally to the tendon with multiple interrupted sutures to prevent splitting of the distal tendon stump.[44,45] This modification can be beneficial if a long distal stump is present (**Fig. 5**).

Synthetic Repair

Fernandez-Fairen and Gimeno performed a series of repairs of Achilles tendon ruptures in athletes using suture augmented with a polyethylene terephthalate mesh synthetic graft. No postoperative immobilization was used. The 29 patients were

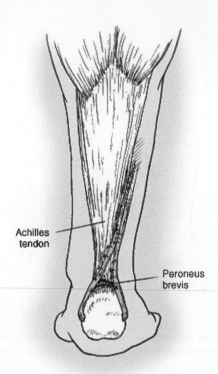

Achilles
tendon

Peroneus
brevis

Fig. 4. Dynamic loop suture of peroneus brevis to itself when end-to-end suture is impossible. (*From* Teuffer AP. Traumatic rupture of the Achilles tendon: reconstruction by transplant and graft using the lateral peroneus brevis. Orthop Clin North Am 1974;5:89–3; with permission.)

aged 25 to 54 years and all practiced sports a minimum of 4 hours weekly. At the follow-up, ranging from 6 months to 5 years, ankle mobility was normal in all but one patient, who had lost 15° of extension. There were no reruptures, although in 2 instances problems with scarring occurred. All patients but one were able to resume their sports activities at the same level of intensity as they had before their injuries.[46] The disadvantage of this repair is that it is voluminous and cordlike when applied to the tendon; consequently problems with healing can occur, or the cord may be perceptible beneath the skin. The augmentation device used is placed across the proximal and distal stumps lateral and medial to the ruptured tendon, and secured to the tendon with absorbable interrupted sutures. The mesh is applied snugly to avoid an increase in volume that might compromise wound healing.

Allograft Augmentation

Several biologic or synthetic scaffolds are being used in Achilles tendon repair, most of them originally developed for use in rotator cuff repair. Barber and colleagues repaired 8 cadaver Achilles tendons by augmenting an end-to-end repair with a human dermal allograft (GraftJacket, Wright Medical Technology, Memphis, TN). These investigators concluded that the load-to-failure of the repair was significantly greater with the augmentation.[47] At present there are only limited reports of clinical experience with the use of these materials for Achilles tendon repair.

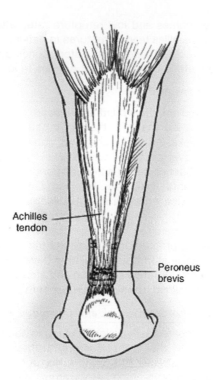

Achilles
tendon

Peroneus
brevis

Fig. 5. Modified peroneus brevis transfer. Peroneus brevis is passed through midcoronal slit in distal stump of Achilles tendon and sutured to stump and to tendon. (*From* Turco VJ, Spinella AJ. Achilles tendon ruptures peroneus brevis transfer. Foot Ankle 1987;7:253–59; with permission. Copyright © 1987 by the American Orthopaedic Foot and Ankle Society Inc.)

REHABILITATION AFTER OPEN REPAIR

The protocols for early postoperative mobilization after repair of Achilles tendon ruptures described in the literature are inconsistent, mostly because of variations in the initiation of weight bearing, the range of motion allowed, and strength training. This inconsistency makes it difficult to determine the importance of each factor in the early rehabilitation process for optimizing recovery. Aoki and colleagues reported no reruptures in 22 athletes treated with primary end-to-end repair, followed by early active motion and partial weight bearing, with full weight bearing at 16 days and return to sport at an average of 13 weeks.[23] All 64 patients reported by Sorrenti resumed their normal activities within an average of 3 months after open repair and early mobilization; however, there were 13 (20%) wound infections.[18] Five randomized controlled trials comparing an early functional rehabilitation protocol with an immobilization protocol all found that early mobilization improved at least one aspect of recovery, such as an earlier return to normal walking and stair-climbing, work, or sports; improved plantar flexion strength; greater range of motion; or reduced calf atrophy.[48–52] Experimental data also have shown that the histologic quality in mobilized tendons is superior to that in immobilized tissue.[53,54] The rehabilitation may actually be more important in determining postoperative function than the method of operative repair. Twaddle and Poon, in a randomized controlled clinical trial, found comparable functional outcomes and low rerupture rates after both operative and nonoperative treatment of Achilles tendon ruptures in patients who followed an early motion rehabilitation protocol.[55] These investigators concluded that early motion is more important that the method of treatment of Achilles tendon ruptures.

Traditional Rehabilitiation Protocol

At 2 weeks, the cast is removed, the wound is inspected, and the staples or sutures are removed. Another short-leg cast with the foot in gravity equinus is worn for an additional 2 weeks. At 4 weeks, the cast is changed, and the foot is gradually brought to the plantigrade position over the next 2 weeks. Walking is gradually resumed with partial weight bearing on crutches during a 2-week period. At 6 to 8 weeks, a removable brace allowing only plantar flexion can be used. Gentle active range-of-motion exercises for 20 minutes twice a day are begun. Isometric ankle exercises along with a knee-strengthening and hip-strengthening program can be instituted. Toe raises, progressive resistance exercises, and proprioceptive exercises, in combination with a general strengthening program, constitute the third stage of rehabilitation. At 12 weeks, a reverse-90° ankle stop brace or similar device is fitted (if not already in use) and is worn until a nearly full range of motion and strength 80% that of the opposite extremity have been obtained, usually within 6 months.

Accelerated Rehabilitation Protocol (Suchak and Colleagues)

Suchak and colleagues compared early weight bearing to nonweight bearing following repair and found that at 6 weeks, the weight-bearing group had significantly better scores and fewer limitations of daily activities. At 6 months, however, no significant differences between the groups were seen in any outcome. No reruptures occurred in either group.[52]

Patients are kept rigidly immobilized with the foot in resting equinus for 2 weeks following surgery. Weight bearing is allowed as tolerated. At 2 weeks, a fixed-angle hinged ankle-foot orthosis (AFO) is applied in resting equinus. Over the next 2 to 3 weeks, the foot is brought into neutral, and active dorsiflexion range-of-motion exercises are done twice a day. At the 6-week postoperative visit, patients are instructed to wean themselves from the use of the AFO as soon as tolerated. Dorsiflexion, plantar flexion, and range-of-motion exercises with resistance tubing; a progressive heel-raise routine; and stationary cycling are added. Exercises are advanced again at the 3-month visit to include unilateral heel raises on the affected leg. At the 6-month postoperative visit, patients are allowed to resume their regular work and recreational activities.

OPEN REPAIR: KEY POINTS

- Early repair (within 7 to 14 days of injury) is optimal.
- Meticulous surgical technique, including gentle soft tissue handling, intraoperative hemostasis, and a layered closure, is essential to avoid wound complications.
- Restoration of normal tendon tension is critical and, in the acute setting, can be obtained by lysis of adhesions or mobilization of the proximal tendon segment.
- Avoiding lengthy immobilization (early mobilization rehabilitation protocol) minimizes recovery time and maximizes function and strength.

SENIOR AUTHOR'S (F.M.A.) PREFERRED METHOD

I prefer to use an open end-to-end repair technique for most patients because of the predictable results and low complication rate. The open technique allows accurate restoration of functional length of the musculotendinous unit, which can be difficult with closed and percutaneous techniques. More complex, 3-bundle and 6-strand suture techniques, though perhaps biomechanically stronger, can be associated with more wound complications because of the bulkiness of the construct, and there is the potential for devascularization of the tendon with multiple complex grasping sutures. I prefer repair with simple Krakow sutures, avoiding knot placement or bulky suture material directly beneath the incision (see **Fig. 1**). The longitudinal medial incision avoids risk of injury to the sural nerve and lesser saphenous venous plexus, and postoperative adhesions are rare with this approach. I prefer to use nonabsorbable nylon sutures to prevent wound-healing problems that can occur with absorbable sutures; these sutures are removed 3 weeks after the repair. Usually an adequate primary repair makes augmentation procedures unnecessary, avoiding the potential for more wound complications; however, if the plantaris is in good condition, I use it for augmentation. An accelerated rehabilitation program is followed (as described earlier), but instead of an AFO, a walking boot with a lift is used.

REFERENCES

1. Maffulli N. Rupture of the Achilles tendon. J Bone Joint Surg Am 1999;81: 1019–36.
2. Lagergren C, Lindholm A. Vascular distribution in the Achilles tendon; an angiographic and microangiographic study. Acta Chir Scand 1959;116:491–5.
3. Viidik A. Tensile strength properties of Achilles tendon systems in trained and untrained rabbits. Acta Orthop Scand 1969;40:261–72.
4. Schepsis AA, Jones H, Haas AL. Achilles tendon disorders in athletes. Am J Sports Med 2002;30:287–305.
5. Saltzman CL, Tearse DS. Achilles tendon injuries. J Am Acad Orthop Surg 1998;6: 316–25.
6. Pare A. Les oeuvres. Lyon (France): Claude Rigaud and Claude Obert; 1633.
7. Lea RB, Smith L. Non-surgical treatment of tendo achillis rupture. J Bone Joint Surg Am 1972;54:1398–407.
8. Nistor L. Surgical and non-surgical treatment of Achilles tendon rupture. A prospective randomized study. J Bone Joint Surg Am 1981;63:394–9.
9. Gillies H, Chalmers J. The management of fresh ruptures of the tendo achillis. J Bone Joint Surg Am 1970;52:337–43.
10. Kellam JF, Hunter GA, McElwain JP. Review of the operative treatment of Achilles tendon rupture. Clin Orthop Relat Res 1985;201:80–3.
11. Bhandari M, Guyatt GH, Siddiqui F, et al. Treatment of acute Achilles tendon ruptures: a systematic overview and metaanalysis. Clin Orthop Relat Res 2002; 400:190–200.
12. Khan RJ, Fick D, Keogh A, et al. Treatment of acute achilles tendon ruptures. A meta-analysis of randomized, controlled trials. J Bone Joint Surg Am 2005; 87:2202–10.
13. Kocher MS, Bishop J, Marshall R, et al. Operative versus nonoperative management of acute Achilles tendon rupture: expected-value decision analysis. Am J Sports Med 2002;30:783–90.
14. Pajala A, Kangas J, Ohtonen P, et al. Rerupture and deep infection following treatment of total Achilles tendon rupture. J Bone Joint Surg Am 2002;84: 2016–21.
15. Scott WN, Inglis AE, Sculco TP. Surgical treatment of reruptures of the tendoachilles following nonsurgical treatment. Clin Orthop Relat Res 1979;140:175–7.

16. Cetti R, Christensen SE, Ejsted R, et al. Operative versus nonoperative treatment of Achilles tendon rupture. A prospective randomized study and review of the literature. Am J Sports Med 1993;21:791–9.
17. Jacobs D, Martens M, Van Audekercke R, et al. Comparison of conservative and operative treatment of Achilles tendon rupture. Am J Sports Med 1978;6:107–11.
18. Sorrenti SJ. Achilles tendon rupture: effect of early mobilization in rehabilitation after surgical repair. Foot Ankle Int 2006;27:407–10.
19. Rettig AC, Liotta FJ, Klootwyk TE, et al. Potential risks of rerupture in primary achilles tendon repair in athletes younger than 30 years of age. Am J Sports Med 2005;33:119–23.
20. Wong J, Barrass V, Maffulli N. Quantitative review of operative and nonoperative management of achilles tendon ruptures. Am J Sports Med 2002;30:565–75.
21. Inglis AE, Sculco TP. Surgical repair of ruptures of the tendo Achillis. Clin Orthop Relat Res 1981;156:160–9.
22. Carden DG, Noble J, Chalmers J, et al. Rupture of the calcaneal tendon. The early and late management. J Bone Joint Surg Br 1987;69:416–20.
23. Aoki M, Ogiwara N, Ohta T, et al. Early active motion and weightbearing after cross-stitch Achilles tendon repair. Am J Sports Med 1998;26:794–800.
24. Jaakkola JI, Hutton WC, Beskin JL, et al. Achilles tendon rupture repair: biomechanical comparison of the triple bundle technique versus the Krakow locking loop technique. Foot Ankle Int 2000;21:14–7.
25. Beskin JL, Sanders RA, Hunter SC, et al. Surgical repair of Achilles tendon ruptures. Am J Sports Med 1987;15:1–8.
26. Akgun U, Erol B, Karahan M [Primary surgical repair with the Krackow technique combined with plantaris tendon augmentation in the treatment of acute Achilles tendon ruptures] Acta Orthop Traumatol Turc 2006;40:228–33.
27. Lennox DW, Wang GJ, McCue FC, et al. The operative treatment of Achilles tendon injuries. Clin Orthop Relat Res 1980;148:152–5.
28. Jessing P, Hansen E. Surgical treatment of 102 tendo achillis ruptures—suture or tenontoplasty? Acta Chir Scand 1975;141:370–7.
29. Levy M, Velkes S, Goldstein J, et al. A method of repair for Achilles tendon ruptures without cast immobilization. Preliminary report. Clin Orthop Relat Res 1984;187:199–204.
30. Lieberman JR, Lozman J, Czajka J, et al. Repair of Achilles tendon ruptures with Dacron vascular graft. Clin Orthop Relat Res 1988;234:204–8.
31. Cetti R, Christensen SE. Surgical treatment under local anesthesia of Achilles tendon rupture. Clin Orthop Relat Res 1983;173:204–8.
32. Keller J, Bak B. The use of anesthesia for surgical treatment of Achilles tendon rupture. Orthopedics 1989;12:431–3.
33. Andersen E, Hvass I. Suture of Achilles tendon rupture under local anesthesia. Acta Orthop Scand 1986;57:235–6.
34. Boyden EM, Kitaoka HB, Cahalan TD, et al. Late versus early repair of Achilles tendon rupture. Clinical and biomechanical evaluation. Clin Orthop Relat Res 1995;317:150–8.
35. Saxena A, Maffulli N, Nguyen A, et al. Wound complications from surgeries pertaining to the Achilles tendon: an analysis of 219 surgeries. J Am Podiatr Med Assoc 2008;98:95–101.
36. Bruggeman NB, Turner NS, Dahm DL, et al. Wound complications after open Achilles tendon repair: an analysis of risk factors. Clin Orthop Relat Res 2004;427:63–6.
37. Ralston EL, Schmidt ER Jr. Repair of the ruptured Achilles tendon. J Trauma 1971; 11:15–21.

38. Fierro NL, Sallis RE. Achilles tendon rupture. Is casting enough? Postgrad Med 1995;98:145–52.
39. Gillespie HS, George EA. Results of surgical repair of spontaneous rupture of the Achilles tendon. J Trauma 1969;9:247–9.
40. DeLee J, Drez D, Miller MD. DeLee & Drez's orthopaedic sports medicine: principles and practice. 2nd edition. Philadelphia: Saunders; 2003.
41. McKeon BP, Heming JF, Fulkerson J, et al. The Krackow stitch: a biomechanical evaluation of changing the number of loops versus the number of sutures. Arthroscopy 2006;22:33–7.
42. Lee SJ, Goldsmith S, Nicholas SJ, et al. Optimizing Achilles tendon repair: effect of epitendinous suture augmentation on the strength of Achilles tendon repairs. Foot Ankle Int 2008;29:427–32.
43. Watson TW, Jurist KA, Yang KH, et al. The strength of Achilles tendon repair: an in vitro study of the biomechanical behavior in human cadaver tendons. Foot Ankle Int 1995;16:191–5.
44. Turco V, Spinella AJ. Team physician #2. Peroneus brevis transfer for Achilles tendon rupture in athletes. Orthop Rev 1988;17:822–4, 827–8.
45. Turco VJ, Spinella AJ. Achilles tendon ruptures—peroneus brevis transfer. Foot Ankle 1987;7:253–9.
46. Fernandez-Fairen M, Gimeno C. Augmented repair of Achilles tendon ruptures. Am J Sports Med 1997;25:177–81.
47. Barber FA, McGarry JE, Herbert MA, et al. A biomechanical study of Achilles tendon repair augmentation using GraftJacket matrix. Foot Ankle Int 2008;29:329–33.
48. Costa ML, Shepstone L, Darrah C, et al. Immediate full-weight-bearing mobilisation for repaired Achilles tendon ruptures: a pilot study. Injury 2003;34:874–6.
49. Cetti R, Henriksen LO, Jacobsen KS. A new treatment of ruptured Achilles tendons. A prospective randomized study. Clin Orthop Relat Res 1994;308:155–65.
50. Kangas J, Pajala A, Siira P, et al. Early functional treatment versus early immobilization in tension of the musculotendinous unit after Achilles rupture repair: a prospective, randomized, clinical study. J Trauma 2003;54:1171–80 [discussion: 1180–1].
51. Mandelbaum BR, Myerson MS, Forster R. Achilles tendon ruptures. A new method of repair, early range of motion, and functional rehabilitation. Am J Sports Med 1995;23:392–5.
52. Suchak AA, Bostick GP, Beaupre LA, et al. The influence of early weight-bearing compared with non-weight-bearing after surgical repair of the Achilles tendon. J Bone Joint Surg Am 2008;90:1876–83.
53. Murrell GA, Jang D, Deng XH, et al. Effects of exercise on Achilles tendon healing in a rat model. Foot Ankle Int 1998;19:598–603.
54. Solveborn SA, Moberg A. Immediate free ankle motion after surgical repair of acute Achilles tendon ruptures. Am J Sports Med 1994;22:607–10.
55. Twaddle BC, Poon P. Early motion for Achilles tendon ruptures: is surgery important? A randomized, prospective study. Am J Sports Med 2007;35:2033–8.

Chronic Achilles Tendon Ruptures

Thomas G. Padanilam, MD[a,b,*]

KEYWORDS

- Chronic Achilles tendon ruptures
- Neglected Achilles tendon ruptures • Achilles
- Tendon transfers for Achilles
- Treatment of chronic Achilles rupture

The Achilles tendon is formed by the two heads of the gastrocnemius muscle and the soleus muscle. Its functional importance is inferred by the observation that it is the strongest and thickest tendon in the body.[1] Loss of Achilles function causes a significant loss in plantar flexion strength, which in turn can lead to an inability to run, stand on tip toes, play sports, and difficulty climbing stairs.[2] The slightly medial to midline insertion on the calcaneal tuberosity creates both an equinus and inversion force.[1]

The Achilles is among the most frequently ruptured tendons.[3] Achilles tendon ruptures are usually seen in the middle-aged male who participates in athletic activities on a recreational basis. These injuries usually present with no significant warning and can cause a sharp pain in the posterior calf area. Patients will often have a sensation of having been "kicked" or "hit" in the calf area. Some patients may hear an audible snap.[4]

Some of these patients, after their initial episode of discomfort, may have significant decrease in their level of pain leading to delays in them seeking medical attention. More commonly, delays in treatment are result of patients presenting for treatment and being misdiagnosed.[5-7] Scheller and colleagues[8] noted that Achilles tendon rupture was missed on the initial evaluation of 25% of their patients. Nesterson and colleagues[9] also reported 25% incidence of missed ruptures on initial evaluation. Inglis and colleagues[10] attributed the 22% of misdiagnoses in their series to physicians and patients being misled by the inconsequential nature of the trauma reported, lack of significant pain, and patient's ability to weakly plantar flex the ankle. Swelling can make a gap difficult to appreciate and action of the long toe flexor may provide enough strength to convince a physician that only a partial rupture has occurred.[8] The plantar flexion weakness seen with most ruptures may be attributed to pain rather than a complete rupture.[7] Significant fraying or shredding of the tendon can also make it difficult to appreciate a palpable gap.[5]

[a] University of Toledo, Toledo, OH 43615, USA
[b] Toledo Orthopaedic Surgeons, 2865 North Reynolds Road, Building A, Toledo, OH 43615, USA
* Toledo Orthopaedic Surgeons, 2865 North Reynolds Road, Building A, Toledo, OH 43615, USA
E-mail address: tgpadanilam@msn.com

Foot Ankle Clin N Am 14 (2009) 711–728
doi:10.1016/j.fcl.2009.08.001
1083-7515/09/$ – see front matter © 2009 Elsevier Inc. All rights reserved.

foot.theclinics.com

Those patients who sustain undiagnosed Achilles ruptures may go on to be considered chronic or neglected ruptures. The transition from what is considered an acute rupture to a chronic rupture is somewhat arbitrary and variable.[2,11,12] The time frame within which an alteration in surgical techniques is required or when patient outcomes vary from acute Achilles ruptures is not well defined. There appears to be some consensus that patients diagnosed 4 to 6 weeks from injury would be classified as a chronic rupture.[2,10,11,13–15] Boyden and colleagues[16] performed a retrospective study comparing outcomes between patients who underwent surgical repair early and those who were treated more than 4 weeks from injury. They performed a fascial turndown flap for augmentation in most of their patients in both groups. They found comparable results between the two groups based on cybex testing. Inglis and colleagues'[10] retrospective review compared outcomes in patient treated within 4 weeks after injury and those after 4 weeks. Inglis and colleagues[10] noted similar outcomes in regards to power and strength between the two groups but noted that the chronic group had 20% less endurance than the acute group. These studies may be compromised by the use of prolonged immobilization in both groups and lack of well-defined rehabilitation protocols. Early mobilization and rehabilitation may improve outcomes seen in the acute rupture setting.[17] There also appears to be a general consensus that the treatment of chronic Achilles ruptures can be more difficult than acute ruptures.[2,11,14,18–20]

PATHOPHYSIOLOGY

An Achilles tendon rupture will trigger a reparative response. Carden and colleagues[21] noted that within 1 week enough granulation tissue will have developed between tendon ends to prevent their apposition in a closed manner. Over time, fibrous tissue will develop in the rupture site.[22–26] Contraction of calf muscles leads to a gradual stretching of this fibrous tissue as it lacks the strength of a normal tendon.[15] The tendon may occasionally heal in continuity in an elongated position with a thickened tendon (**Fig. 1**).[25,27] The elongation of the tendon leads to loss in the mechanical efficiency of the triceps surae complex. Elftman[28] noted that ability of muscle fibers to produce tension will decrease as the muscle fibers shorten and will become almost zero when the muscle fibers approximate 60% of resting length. This leads to ankle plantar flexion weakness and its associated gait disturbances. The continued contraction of the triceps surae muscle will more commonly lead to retraction of the proximal tendon stump leading to a gap between the ruptured ends.[15,20,29,30] The magnitude of

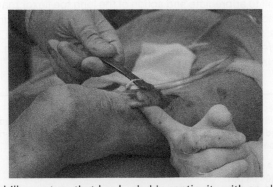

Fig. 1. A chronic Achilles rupture that has healed in continuity with an elongated tendon.

the gap can be variable and the associated retraction of the proximal tendon can prevent end-to-end apposition of tendon. In addition, it can be difficult to identify a separate tendon sheath and proximal stump can be adhered to the posterior fascia (**Fig. 2**).[30] The plantaris tendon, when it is present, may be hypertrophied.[2] In chronic ruptures, the Achilles tendon will often appear dull in appearance, irregular in shape, and be adherent to the surrounding fascia.[19]

PATIENT EVALUATION

Patients with chronic or neglected Achilles tendon rupture may present with symptoms that are vague and not necessarily localized to the Achilles tendon region. Pain the Achilles area is often not what causes the patient to seek medical attention. This lack of sharp discomfort in the Achilles region may contribute to delays in diagnosis. Patients may notice swelling around the ankle. They will often complain of a sense of fatigue or weakness with prolonged ambulation.[12] This can also be characterized as a sense of unsteadiness in their gait. Patients may report difficulty climbing stairs and walking uphill. They may also complain of an inability to get up onto their toes.[9,12,31]

On examination, patients will usually show signs of calf atrophy or wasting. Patients may show a calcaneous gait with loss of normal push-off.[32] The Achilles tendon often loses its normal contour. There may be a visible defect around the tendon or if a significant scar response has occurred there may be the appearance of fullness around the tendon. Those patients with a visible defect may develop a skin contracture around the rupture, which may need to be considered when developing a treatment plan.

The presence of a palpable gap can be variable. Some patients will have retraction of the proximal end of the rupture with minimal reparative tissue between the rupture ends or if reparative response did occur the tissue may elongate and attenuate over time. These patients will have a palpable gap. In others the reparative process can lead to tissue filling the gap to the point that no palpable gap is appreciated between the ends.

The rupture will lead to increased passive dorsiflexion of the ankle as the normal Achilles tendon restraint is lost. There is usually plantar flexion weakness and most patients are unable to perform a single leg heel raise. Occasionally, patients will

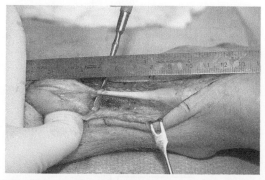

Fig. 2. Chronic rupture with retraction of the proximal tendon leading to a gap between the two ends of the tendon. The plantaris tendon has hypertrophied and is shown crossing the rupture site. The tip of the freer shows the proximal tendon stump scarred down to the tendon sheath.

have sufficient strength in the other plantar flexors that they are able to perform a single leg heel raise but are usually unable to perform multiple or repetitive heel raises.[15]

The Thompson or Simmonds test has been used to detect Achilles tendon ruptures. This was first described by Simmonds[5] and popularized by Thompson and Doherty.[33] The test is performed by the patient lying prone with feet hanging over the edge of the examining table. The calf squeeze causes a lifting of the gastrocnemius, which in turn causes a shortening of the Achilles tendon.[6] This shortening causes a plantar flexion response in the foot. Failure of the foot to move into plantar flexion is considered diagnostic of an Achilles tendon rupture. Maffulli[13] noted that in cases of acute ruptures this test is highly reliable. In chronic cases, the reliability of this test may be reduced such that the presence of plantar flexion of the foot may not indicate an intact Achilles tendon.[24,32] Thompson and Doherty[33] noted that in chronic ruptures the tendon may scar down to surrounding structures leading to a weak plantar flexion response. Plantar flexion of the foot may also be caused by organization of hematoma over time leading to some continuity in the tendon.[13]

Matles[32] described a test for evaluating Achilles tendon ruptures. Patients are placed in a prone position with the foot over the edge of the bed. The patient is asked to actively flex the knee to 90 degrees. Active flexion of the knee should cause the gastrocnemius to shorten leading to plantar flexion of the foot. If the foot falls into neutral or slight dorsiflexion, the Achilles tendon is considered to be ruptured. In chronic ruptures, elongation of the tendon or loss of continuity can lead to a positive test (**Fig. 3**).

Two other examination findings that can aid in the diagnosis of Achilles ruptures have been described by O'Brien[6] and Copeland.[7] The O'Brien test is performed with the patient prone and a needle inserted through the skin of the calf at a right angle just medial to the midline at a point about 10 cm above the calcaneal insertion of the tendon. The needle is inserted until further resistance is felt and needle tip is within the

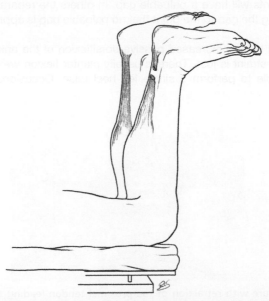

Fig. 3. A positive Matles test. Flexion of knee causes the leg with an Achilles rupture or tendon that has healed in an elongated fashion to assume a more dorsiflexed position. (*Courtesy of* Toledo Orthopaedic Surgeons, Toledo, OH; with permission.)

substance of the tendon without transfixing the tendon. The ankle is passively dorsi-flexed and if the tendon is intact, the tip of the needle will point proximally. The Cope-land test is performed with the patient prone and a blood pressure cuff placed around the mid-calf. The cuff is inflated to 100 mm Hg with the foot in plantar flexion. The foot is then passively dorsiflexed. If the pressure rises to 140 mm Hg, the Achilles tendon is presumed to be intact. Failure of the pressure to change indicates a rupture of the tendon. The O'Brien and Copeland tests were described for use in the acute setting; however, their value or role in the chronic rupture situation has not been well studied or established.

Imaging studies may also aid in the diagnosis of chronic Achilles ruptures. Radio-graphs may reveal an avulsion of the Achilles tendon from its calcaneal insertion. In addition, calcification may be seen within the proximal stump of the tendon.[34] Real-time high-resolution ultrasound may be helpful in the diagnosis in that it can reveal an acoustic vacuum at the rupture site with the presence of thick irregular edges.[14] Difficulty in using ultrasound relates to it being highly user dependent and need for significant experience to correctly interpret the images.[31]

Magnetic resonance imaging can be helpful in the evaluation of patients with Achilles tendon injuries.[35] The normal Achilles tendon is seen as a low-intensity band on all sequences. Chronic ruptures can be seen as an area of low-intensity signal on T1-weighted images and alteration in T2-weighted signal (**Fig. 4**).[31] It can be useful in providing an estimation of the gap between the ruptured ends.

TREATMENT OPTIONS

Management of patients with chronic Achilles ruptures involves both operative and nonoperative options. The choice between these options should made after taking into consideration the overall health status of the patient, assessment of risk factors

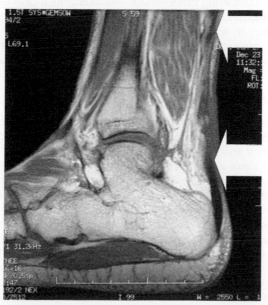

Fig. 4. An MRI image with white arrows pointing to the ends of the Achilles tendon ends. The area between the arrows represents the gap between the tendon ends.

for healing, and the patient's level of activity. Christensen[36] reported on a retrospective series with 57 Achilles tendon ruptures, most of which were chronic. The author used inability to perform a single leg heel raise as an indication for surgery. Management in 18 of 57 ruptures consisted of observation only, whereas the other 39 were treated surgically. The author found that, based on Achilles function and pain as criteria, the operative group showed 90% improvement whereas the nonoperative group showed a 70% improvement. Only 56% of patients in the nonoperative group had restored function, whereas 75% in the operative group did. The author noted that with nonoperative treatment improvement may take years and can be accompanied by period of pain until healing is complete.

Nonoperative treatment can be considered for those patients who have associated comorbidities, such as peripheral vascular disease, which makes them poor surgical candidates. Nonoperative treatment is also indicated for those patients who do not have any significant functional deficits and are able to perform their activities of daily living.[15] These typically are patients who have a relatively sedentary lifestyle that can accommodate the loss of strength associated with Achilles rupture. The use of a molded ankle foot orthosis (AFO) with or without a hinge may be helpful. Some patients tolerate the brace well and notice improvement in regard to stability of the leg.[15] I have found that patients, for whom nonoperative treatment is indicated, may benefit from a structured rehabilitation program to strengthen the remaining flexor muscles to help partially compensate for loss of Achilles function.

Although nonoperative treatment may be indicated for some patients with chronic ruptures, most patients are best managed with surgical reconstruction.[2,10,11,14,18,19,26,29,34,37–39] There have been a variety of methods described as being effective in reconstruction of chronic Achilles tendon ruptures.[1,10,18–20,22,26,29,30,34,37–41] The main objective of surgical treatment is to restore the normal length and tension to the Achilles tendon complex.[8,42] Kangas and colleagues[43] noted that patients with greater elongation of their tendon after repair had worse clinical outcomes. There is very little to no data comparing these various methods of treatment used in reconstruction of chronic Achilles tendon ruptures. Before proceeding with any type of surgical intervention it is important to address associated comorbidities such as smoking, chronic swelling, and any associated skin contracture. Some patients may require the use of tissue expanders to allow tension-free wound closure after the reconstruction.[12]

TENDON INCONTINUITY

Some patients with chronic ruptures will not have any significant gap between the two ends of the rupture.[15] There is lengthening of the Achilles tendon leading to a loss in its mechanical efficiency and subsequent loss of power. The tendon may appear intact on exploration but there is evidence of scarring in the tendon sheath. Maffulli and Ajis[31] described performing a z-shortening in this group of patients to restore the resting length of the gastro-soleus complex by placing the ankle in slightly greater equinus than on the contralateral side.

Porter and colleagues[27] reported on a series of 11 patients treated 4 to 12 weeks from the time of rupture. They circumferentially freed the two tendon ends and freshened the ends by removing 2 to 4 mm of fibrous scar tissue. They found an average gap of 3 to 5 cm between the tendon ends once the tendon ends were freshened and before the proximal release. The tendon ends were able to be opposed once they were freed up and existing fibrinous scar was used as local reconstruction tissue. The tendon was repaired with the ankle in 20 to 30 degrees of plantar flexion. Porter and colleagues[27] also performed a biopsy of the scar tissue and found the presence of vascular granulation tissue within the rupture site. They noted that with increasing time from injury to surgery, there was a decreasing degree of vascularity within the biopsy specimens. Patients in this study were noted to have an average 8.6% decrease in strength on the operative side, which did not limit participation in sports. Most patients had no subjective weakness and did not have much discomfort with sporting activities. All patients in this study were treated within 12 weeks from injury and thus represent a subset of patients with chronic Achilles tendon ruptures. The time frame after which the vascularity in the fibrinous tissue will no longer support this approach is unknown. Yasuda and colleagues[25] also used this approach in the treatment of six patients and reported similar findings. They correlated the histology at the rupture site with a preoperative MRI and reported that patients whose T2 or gradient echo images showed the tendon to be thickened and fusiform in shape with diffuse intratendinous high signal changes could be treated with this approach. If the MRI showed a tendon that was narrowed with focal high signal changes, then another method of reconstruction should be used.[25]

TENDON MOBILIZATION

A long-standing rupture more commonly results in a gap between the rupture ends.[15] The continued contraction of the gastro-soleus complex leads to retraction of the proximal tendon stump. There is considerable variability in the magnitude of the gap between the two ruptured ends. Smaller gaps, such as around 2 cm, can often be repaired with an end-to-end repair.[12,31] Sometimes slightly longer gaps can be closed by the placement of a Krackow stitch and manual traction for several minutes intraoperatively to help stretch the proximal musculature (Fig. 5).[44] This is usually combined with bluntly freeing the tendon ends from the surrounding soft tissues.

TURNDOWN FLAPS

Several different methods of turndown flaps have been described in the treatment of Achilles tendon ruptures. Christensen[36] described the use of a 2 × 10-cm flap that was raised from the proximal tendon fragment and turned down to cover the defect in both acute and chronic ruptures. He reported 75% of outcomes as being satisfactory. Bosworth[22] reported on six patients with chronic ruptures treated with a fascial turndown graft. The technique consisted of removing the fibrous tissue between the two tendon ends followed by freeing up a strip of tendon from the proximal tendon stump (Fig. 6). This strip of tendon is woven through the proximal stump transversely and then through the distal stump of the rupture and finally back again through the proximal stump. This acts as a bridge of tissue connecting the two ruptured ends. Bosworth[22] reported good results in his six patients treated with this technique. Barnes and Hardy[24] studied 11 patients who were treated surgically for chronic ruptures. They reported that 8 of 11 patients were fully satisfied; however, only 1 patient was asymptomatic. The rest of the patients reported mild to moderate stiffness, weakness, and discomfort. Rush[29] raised an inverted "U" from the proximal fascia and then sutured the ends together to create a tube. All five patients were happy and could return to activities; however, they noted some weakness compared with the other side. Arner and Lindholm[45] evaluated three different turndown flaps in their series of patients and found no significant functional difference among the various techniques. Maffulli and Leadbetter[42] noted that the quality of the proximal stump is often suboptimal for the use of a turndown flap. These techniques are essentially using avascular autologous tissue to fill the gap between ends of a chronic rupture.

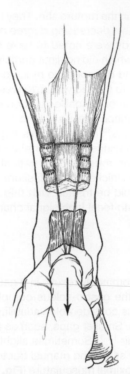

Fig. 5. Placement of a Krackow stitch in the proximal Achilles tendon and application of manual traction. Application of traction over several minutes will allow stretching of the muscle and decrease the gap between the tendon ends. (*Courtesy of* Toledo Orthopaedic Surgeons, Toledo, OH; with permission.)

TENDON ADVANCEMENT

Abraham and Pankovich[20] described the use of a V-Y tendinous flap for the end-to-end repair of chronic Achilles ruptures. They adopted this technique as a result of poor experiences using fascial turndown flaps and fascia lata transfers. They found these procedures led to adhesions at the repair site to the overlying skin and weakness of calf muscles, which resulted in poor push-off strength. They reported results in four patients with chronic Achilles rupture, with a gap of 5 to 6 cm between ends, with three of four patients regaining full strength. The length of the gap was measured with the knee in 30 degrees of flexion and the ankle in 20 degrees of plantar flexion. Their procedure involved placing the apex of an inverted "V" incision over central part of the proximal aponeurosis (**Fig. 7**). The arms of the "V" incision should be 1.5 times the length of the gap to be able to close the proximal portion of the aponeurosis in a "Y" fashion. The arms of the incision have to extend through the aponeurosis and the underlying muscle tissue along the sides of the flap. They noted that in some cases it may be necessary to dissect the flap almost completely free to obtain an end-to-end closure of the tendon. The authors speculated that the dissection may render the flap devoid of blood supply, but the flap becomes revascularized either from surrounding tissue or from the paratenon. Myerson[15] has stated that the flap can be advanced to close a gap up to 5 cm and still preserve the posterior muscle attachment. Gaps larger than that may lead to detachment of the posterior muscle group. Leitner and

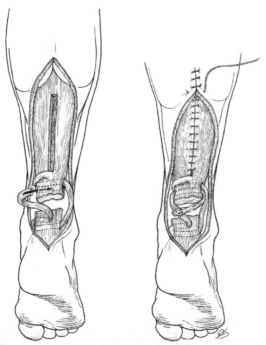

Fig 6. A fascial turndown flap that is harvested from the proximal tendon and weaved through the distal achilles tendon stump. (*Courtesy of* Toledo Orthopaedic Surgeons, Toledo, OH; with permission.)

colleagues[39] reported on three patients who had 8- to 10-cm defects closed with the use of this technique and had good results. Parker and Repinecz[23] in their case report noted that a tendon advancement technique had the advantage of allowing healthy tendon-to-tendon apposition, minimizing tension at the repair site and avoiding foreign materials at the site of healing. Us and colleagues[26] reported on six patients treated with this technique. All six patients were able to perform a single leg heel raise, walk on their toes, and return to preinjury activities. Cybex testing of these patients noted a peak torque deficiency from 2.5% to 22.0% when compared with the contra-lateral limb. They inferred that the V-Y recession allows intrinsic healing resulting in a tendon with enhanced elasticity, strength, and mobility and additionally avoided the sacrifice of other significant lower limb tendons.

TENDON TRANSFERS

The use of the peroneus brevis tendon in the repair of Achilles tendon ruptures was described by Perez-Teuffer.[3] This retrospective study of 30 patients with acute Achilles ruptures described harvesting the tendon from it insertion at the fifth meta-tarsal base and pulling it through to the posterior incision. The tendon was then routed through a drill hole in the calcaneus going from lateral to medial. The tendon was then brought to the proximal Achilles tendon stump and secured to it. The peroneal tendon made a "U"-shaped support around the Achilles tendon. He reported that 28 of 30 had an excellent result and 2 had a good result. Turco and Spinella[1] reported similar results with use of peroneus brevis tendon in the acute setting in 40 patients. They modified

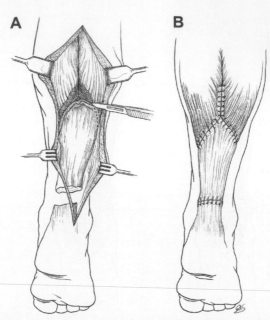

Fig. 7. (*A*) Placement of a inverted "V" in the proximal aponeurosis to close a gap between the ends of a chronic Achilles rupture. (*B*) Advancement of the tendon with closure of the gap and the conversion of the "V" into a "Y" (*Courtesy of* Toledo Orthopaedic Surgeons, Toledo, OH; with permission.)

the technique slightly by placing the peroneus brevis through the distal stump of the Achilles rather than a drill hole in the calcaneus. Most patients were able to return to activities, including sports, without any significant functional limitations. Pintore and colleagues[4] reported on the use of peroneus brevis tendon transfers in 22 patients with chronic Achilles tendon ruptures. They compared outcomes with 59 patients who underwent repair of an acute Achilles rupture. Pintore and colleagues[4] found that although both groups achieved good results, there was a greater tendency for complications and slightly worse functional results in those patients with chronic ruptures. These differences, however, were not statistically different between the two groups. They reported that although the patients did not report any subjective weakness, isokinetic strength testing revealed significantly lower peak torque in patients with chronic ruptures when compared with acute ruptures. They also found that patients with a peroneus brevis transfer had deficiencies in eversion strength; however, no patients reported this as a subjective problem. Whether the loss of eversion strength will lead to any functional problems is unknown. It has also been noted that placement of the peroneus brevis in a lateral to medial direction may fail to duplicate the more medial pull of the Achilles.[34] Use of the peroneus brevis may result in a loss of the normal muscle balance between the invertors and evertors and in addition the use of an evertor to substitute for plantar flexion role of the Achilles may result in a less functional repair.[40]

Mann and colleagues[34] reported on seven patients in whom the flexor digitorum longus (FDL) tendon was used for the reconstruction of chronic Achilles tendon ruptures. The FDL tendon was harvested in the midfoot near the master knot of Henry and brought into the posterior incision. It was passed via a drill hole in the calcaneus from medial to lateral and then tied onto itself. The FDL tendon was tensioned with the foot in 10 to 15 degrees of plantar flexion. In addition, a central turndown flap was used to augment the FDL tendon and was placed into the distal stump or the calcaneus. Mann and colleagues[34] advocated the advantages of the FDL to include avoidance of host rejection, which may be seen with allograft or synthetic materials, does not require revascularization, as seen with free tissue transfer and turndown flap, and that its biomechanical characteristics are similar to the Achilles.

Wapner and colleagues[40] described the use of the flexor hallucis longus (FHL) tendon in the reconstruction of chronic Achilles ruptures. In their study of seven patients, three were reported as having excellent results, three good, and one fair result. All patients were noted to have some loss of flexion of the interphalangeal joint of the hallux, but this was unnoticed by the patients until pointed out to them at follow-up. Surgical positioning for an FHL tendon transfer can be supine, prone, or lateral. Lateral positioning with the affected extremity down and then rolling the patient slightly prone facilitates exposure of both the posterior aspect of the leg and the medial side of the foot (**Fig. 8**). A longitudinal incision is made along the medial aspect of the Achilles centered at the level of the rupture and of sufficient length to allow exposure of the tendon on both ends of the rupture (**Fig. 9**). The incision is carried sharply down to the level of the tendon to maintain as thick a soft tissue envelope as possible around the Achilles. The tendon is often scarred down to the sheath and is usually best identified and separated from the sheath along the proximal aspect. The intervening scar tissue is excised back to healthy tendon. The FHL tendon is identified by opening the fascia over the posterior compartment. The FHL can be harvested from the posterior incision or through a separate incision in the midfoot (**Fig. 10**).[12] Tashjian and colleagues[46] performed a cadaveric study and noted that harvesting the FHL in midfoot at the knot of Henry would provide an average of 3 cm of additional tendon. Tashjian and colleagues[46] questioned whether the additional morbidity of a second incision and added surgical time was worth the unproven benefit of additional graft length. Mulier and colleagues[47] noted the plantar nerves to be at risk with harvesting of the FHL at the midfoot level. In their cadaveric study, 8 of 24 specimens had some degree of injury to either the medial or lateral plantar nerve. Wapner and colleagues[40] harvested the FHL tendon distal to the knot of Henry and noted that an additional 10 to 12 cm of tendon could be obtained for grafting compared with the posterior harvesting of the tendon. This additional length allowed weaving of the tendon through both stumps and may enhance the repair.

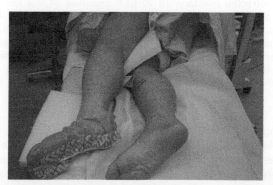

Fig. 8. Lateral positioning with the affected leg down allows access to both the posterior aspect of the leg and medial border of the foot.

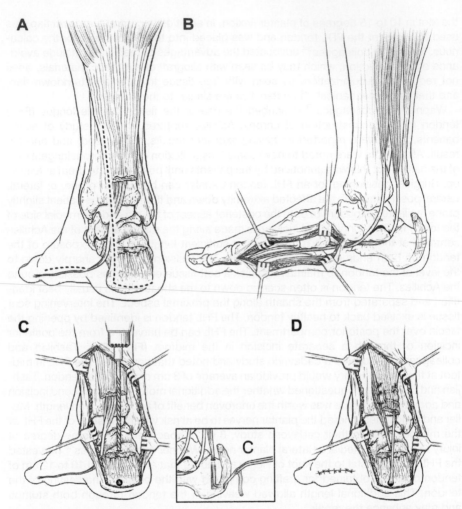

Fig. 9. (*A*) Incision along the posterior-medial aspect of the torn Achilles tendon is shown as well as the medial midfoot incision for harvest of the FHL tendon. (*B*) A medial incision in made from the navicular tuberosity to the first metatarsal. The abductor hallucis and flexor hallucis brevis are retracted plantarward to gain exposure of the FHL tendon. The FHL tendon is released distally and brought into the posterior incision. (*C*) A chronic rupture with a gap between tendon ends. A drill hole is place slightly medial to midline on the calcaneal tuberosity if there is insufficient distal Achilles tendon stump to weave the FHL tendon through. The FHL tendon is then brought superior to posterior through this bone tunnel. (*D*) The FHL tendon is then weaved through the proximal Achilles tendon and secured after passage through the bone tunnel. (*Courtesy of* Toledo Orthopaedic Surgeons, Toledo, OH; with permission.)

Dalal and colleagues[48] noted the FHL tendon transfer to be a low morbidity procedure, for chronic Achilles tendon ruptures, which gave good to excellent results. Wilcox and colleagues[41] reported good to excellent results in their series of patients who underwent FHL tendon transfer for chronic Achilles disorders. Their study showed no complaints regarding the loss of hallux interphalangeal flexion strength. Frenette and Jackson,[49] in their review of young athletes who sustained laceration to the FHL,

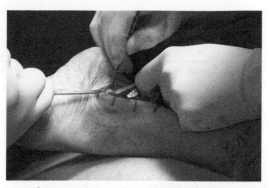

Fig. 10. Proximal harvest of FHL tendon performed through the posterior incision.

concluded that the FHL was not essential for good pushoff and balance in running sports. Coull and colleagues[50] evaluated the postoperative morbidity associated with FHL tendon transfers and noted that all patients had active plantar flexion of the MTP joint but no active IP plantar flexion. No patient had impairment of walking, running, and stair climbing or rising from a crouched position because of weakness of the hallux.

Silver and colleagues[51] noted that the ideal transfer should closely approximate the functional characteristics of the muscle it is replacing without sacrificing any essential function. They calculated the relative contribution of each muscle in the lower leg to the overall strength of the leg. They found that the soleus contributed 29.9% of the strength of the lower extremity whereas the peroneus brevis was 2.6%, FDL was 1.8%, peroneus longus was 5.5%, and the FHL was 3.6%. Based on this, Wapner and colleagues[40] proposed several advantages to the use of FHL for Achilles tendon reconstruction. First is that the FHL is stronger than either the FDL or peroneus brevis. Although the strength of the FHL does not come close to approaching strength of the gastroc-soleus complex, there may be a theoretical advantage in having the additional strength. The FHL contractile axis most closely reproduces that of the Achilles tendon. In addition, the FHL fires in phase with the Achilles, thus maintaining the normal muscle balance around the foot by transferring a plantarflexor to a plantarflexor. Wapner and colleagues[40] also felt the anatomic proximity of the FHL to the Achilles avoids the need to disturb the lateral compartment or the neurovascular bundle. In addition, the distal musculature of the FHL may provide some vascularity to the Achilles tendon.[41]

FREE TISSUE TRANSFER

The use of free tissue transfer has been advocated for bridging the gaps seen in chronic Achilles ruptures. Tobin[19] described the use of fascia lata to address chronic Achilles ruptures in seven patients. He had delayed wound healing in two patients, but otherwise reported good results. Bugg and Boyd[18] treated 10 patients with the use of a sheet of fascia lata from the same or opposite thigh. Three strips were cut from the fascia sheet and weaved into the proximal and distal stump of the Achilles tendon. The remaining sheet was sutured around the strips with the serosal side facing outward. Bugg and Boyd[18] reported satisfactory results with no difficulty with adherent scar. Zadek presented a case report involving the harvest of three strips of fascia from the thigh and weaving them into the tendon ends.[30] He also reported an excellent result with no complications at the donor site. Maffulli and Leadbetter[42] used free

Table 1			
Treatment recommendations for chronic Achilles ruptures			
Myerson[15]	**Kuwada[55]**	**Den Hartog[12]**	**Maffulli and Ajis[31]**
< 2-cm gap - End-to-end repair - Posterior compartment fasciotomy 2–5-cm gap - V-Y lengthening - FHL transfer if gastro muscle not healthy appearing > 5-cm gap - FHL transfer - Can add V-Y advancement to transfer	< 3-cm gap - End-to-end repair 3–6-cm gap - Autogenous tendon flap (turndown flap) - Synthetic graft can be used to augment repair site > 6-cm gap - Gastrocnemius recession - Free tendon and/or synthetic graft	< 2-cm gap - End-to-end repair 2–5-cm gap - Proximal FHL harvest & transfer - Add V-Y or gastrocnemius recession to transfer > 5-cm gap - Proximal FHL harvest & transfer - Add turndown flap > 10-cm gap - Proximal FHL harvest & transfer - Achilles allograft	End-to-end repair when possible - Peroneus brevis transfer when end-to-end not possible - FDL transfer if gap too large for peroneus brevis - Avoid synthetic grafts - Gracilis or semitendinosus autografts for gaps >6.5 cm and local viable tendons not enough

gracilis tendon grafts for chronic Achilles ruptures. This study had 21 patients with an average gap of 6 to 8 cm with the ankle in maximum plantar flexion and tension applied to the proximal Achilles tendon stump. The gracilis tendon was harvested and weaved through both stumps of the Achilles tendon. Superficial wound infection was noted in 5 of 21 patients. All patients were able to return to work and resumed preinjury activities by 2 years postoperatively.

The use of Achilles tendon allograft has also been described in chronic ruptures.[52,53] The allogeneic tissue acts as cellular scaffold for the migration of host cells.[52] The advantages of allograft include the avoidance of morbidity from autogenous autograft, the quality and amount of autogenous tendon may be insufficient to reconstruct Achilles, decreased operative time from not having to perform a harvest, and excellent mechanical properties.[53] The disadvantages to allograft include the potential risk of disease transmission and the high cost associated with purchase of the allograft. Although the use of allograft tissue has been described, I am unaware of any studies with significant numbers that have detailed its efficacy.

SYNTHETIC GRAFTS

A variety of synthetic materials have been used to restore continuity to the Achilles tendon. Jennings and Sefton[37] recommended the use of polyester tape as a synthetic graft for filling defects found with chronic Achilles ruptures. The tape was weaved through the proximal tendon and the calcaneus with tension applied to the proximal stump. The tape was designed to allow formation of scar tissue within the gap. Jennings and Sefton's[37] study of 16 patients noted some weakness compared with the normal side but most patients were noted to have thickening of the tendon with minimal symptoms. Howard and colleagues[54] used carbon fiber weaved through either the calcaneus or distal stump of the tendon to fill the gap. All five patients in the study achieved excellent results and four of five were able to return to preinjury activity level. Ozaki and colleagues[38] used a polypropylene mesh in chronic ruptures and reported satisfactory function at follow-up. Most of the reports regarding the use of synthetic grafts have small numbers of patients, making a comparative evaluation difficult. There is some concern regarding using a nonabsorbable material in an area prone to wound breakdown or infection.[42]

TREATMENT ALGORITHMS

Myerson,[15] Den Hartog,[12] Mafulli,[31] Ajis[31] and Kuwada[55] have proposed treatment algorithms based on the magnitude of the gap seen at surgery (see **Table 1**).[12,15,31,55] Although most studies report the presence of a gap and provide some representation of the magnitude of the gap, there does not appear to be any standardization in regard to how this measurement was obtained. In addition, the algorithms represent expert opinion, as there is a lack of comparative data that can be used to make firm recommendations.

SUMMARY

Chronic Achilles tendon ruptures can be challenging to treat. Most of these are a result of failure to make the initial diagnosis. Although pain is not a prominent symptom, these patients have significant functional deficits that can interfere with activities of daily living. Nonoperative treatment options are limited and probably best reserved for patients with low functional demands or those with significant medical contraindications for surgical treatment. Surgical treatment of chronic rupture often involves the need to restore continuity to tendon ends that may have retracted leading to irreducible gaps. A variety of techniques have been described to address this situation. Most of the reports have shown improvement in patient outcomes with surgical intervention; however, most patients continue to show some strength deficits in comparison to their contralateral limb. The small number of patients in these studies combined with variations in patient selection, postoperative regimens, and outcome measurements make meaningful comparisons difficult. Restoration of the physiologic tension of the gastrocnemius-soleus complex is the goal of surgical intervention and controlled studies are needed to determine if one method is superior to others in the achievement of this goal.

REFERENCES

1. Turco VJ, Spinella AJ. Achilles tendon ruptures—peroneus brevis transfer. Foot Ankle 1987;7:253–9.
2. Leslie H, Edwards W. Neglected ruptures of Achilles tendon. Foot Ankle Clin 2005;10:357–70.
3. Perez-Teuffer A. Traumatic rupture of the Achilles tendon. Reconstruction by transplant and graft using the lateral peroneus brevis. Orthop Clin North Am 1974;5:89–93.
4. Pintore E, Barra V, Pintore R, et al. Peroneus brevis tendon transfer in neglected tears of the Achilles tendon. J Trauma 2001;50:71–8.
5. Simmonds FA. The diagnosis of the ruptured Achilles tendon. Practitioner 1957; 179:56–8.
6. O'Brien T. The needle test for complete rupture of the Achilles tendon. J Bone Joint Surg Am 1984;66:1099–101.

7. Copeland SA. Rupture of the Achilles tendon: a new clinical test. Ann R Coll Surg Engl 1990;72:270–1.
8. Scheller A, Kasser J, Quigley T. Tendon injuries about the ankle. Orthop Clin North Am 1980;11:801–11.
9. Nestorson J, Movin T, Moller M, et al. Function after Achilles tendon rupture in the elderly: 25 patients older than 65 years followed for 3 years. Acta Orthop Scand 2000;71:64–8.
10. Inglis AE, Scott WN, Sculco TP, et al. Ruptures of the tendo Achillis. An objective assessment of surgical and non-surgical treatment. J Bone Joint Surg Am 1976; 58:990–3.
11. Gabel S, Manoli A II. Neglected rupture of the Achilles tendon. Foot Ankle Int 1994;15:512–7.
12. Den Hartog B. Surgical strategies: delayed diagnosis or neglected Achilles' tendon ruptures. Foot Ankle Int 2008;29:456–63.
13. Maffulli N. The clinical diagnosis of subcutaneous tear of the Achilles tendon. A prospective study in 174 patients. Am J Sports Med 1998;26:266–70.
14. Maffulli N, Ajis A, Longo UG, et al. Chronic rupture of tendo Achillis. Foot Ankle Clin N Am 2007;12:583–96.
15. Myerson MS. Achilles tendon ruptures. Instr Course Lect 1999;48:219–30.
16. Boyden EM, Kitaoka HB, Cahalan TD, et al. Late versus early repair of Achilles tendon rupture. Clinical and biomechanical evaluation. Clin Orthop Relat Res 1995;317:150–8.
17. Mandelbaum BR, Myerson MS, Forster R. Achilles tendon ruptures: a new method of repair, early range of motion, and functional rehabilitation. Am J Sports Med 1995;23:392–5.
18. Bugg El Jr, Boyd BM. Repair of neglected rupture or laceration of the Achilles tendon. Clin Orthop Relat Res 1968;56:73–5.
19. Tobin WJ. Repair of the neglected ruptured and severed Achilles tendon. Am Surg 1953;19:514–22.
20. Abraham E, Pankovich AM. Neglected rupture of the Achilles tendon. Treatment by V-Y tendinous flap. J Bone Joint Surg Am 1975;57:253–5.
21. Carden DG, Noble J, Chalmers J, et al. Rupture of the calcaneal tendon. The early and late management. J Bone Joint Surg Br 1987;69:416–20.
22. Bosworth DM. Repair of defects in the tendo Achillis. J Bone Joint Surg Am 1956; 38:111–4.
23. Parker RG, Repinecz M. Neglected rupture of the Achilles tendon. Treatment by modified Strayer gastrocnemius recession. J Am Podiatry Assoc 1979;69: 548–55.
24. Barnes MJ, Hardy AE. Delayed reconstruction of the calcaneal tendon. J Bone Joint Surg Br 1986;68:121–4.
25. Yasuda T, Kinoshita M, Okuda R. Reconstruction of chronic Achilles tendon rupture with the use of interposed tissue between the stumps. Am J Sports Med 2007;35:582–8.
26. Us AK, Bilgin SS, Aydin T, et al. Repair of neglected Achilles tendon ruptures: procedures and functional results. Arch Orthop Trauma Surg 1997;116:408–11.
27. Porter DA, Mannarino FP, Snead D, et al. Primary repair without augmentation for early neglected Achilles tendon ruptures in the recreational athlete. Foot Ankle Int 1997;18:557–64.
28. Elftman H. Biomechanics of muscle with particular application to studies of gait. J Bone Joint Surg Am 1966;48:363–77.

29. Rush JH. Operative repair of neglected rupture of the tendo Achillis. Aust N Z J Surg 1980;50:420–2.
30. Zadek I. Repair of old rupture of the tendo-Achilles by means of fascia. Report of a case. J Bone Joint Surg 1940;22:1070–1.
31. Maffulli N, Ajis A. Management of chronic ruptures of the Achilles tendon. J Bone Joint Surg Am 2008;90:1348–60.
32. Matles AL. Rupture of the tendo Achilles. Another diagnostic sign. Bull Hosp Joint Dis 1975;36:48–51.
33. Thompson TC, Doherty J. Spontaneous rupture of tendon of Achilles: a new clinical diagnostic test. J Trauma 1962;2:126–9.
34. Mann RA, Holmes GB Jr, Seale KS, et al. Chronic rupture of the Achilles tendon: a new technique of repair. J Bone Joint Surg Am 1991;73:214–9.
35. Karjalainen P, Hannu A, Pihlajamaki H, et al. Magnetic resonance imaging during healing of surgically repaired Achilles tendon ruptures. Am J Sports Med 1997; 25:164–71.
36. Christensen I. Rupture of the Achilles tendon: analysis of 57 cases. Acta Chir Scand 1953;106:50–60.
37. Jennings AG, Sefton GK. Chronic rupture of tendo Achillis. Long-term results of operative management using polyester tape. J Bone Joint Surg Br 2002;84: 361–3.
38. Ozaki J, Fujiki J, Sugimoto K, et al. Reconstruction of neglected Achilles tendon rupture with Marlex mesh. Clin Orthop Relat Res 1989;238:204–8.
39. Leitner A, Voigt C, Rahmanzadeh R. Treatment of extensive aseptic defects in old Achilles tendon ruptures: methods and case reports. Foot Ankle 1992;13:176–80.
40. Wapner KL, Pavlock GS, Hecht PJ, et al. Repair of chronic Achilles tendon rupture with flexor hallucis longus tendon transfer. Foot Ankle 1993;14:443–9.
41. Wilcox DK, Bohay DR, Anderson JG. Treatment of chronic Achilles tendon disorders with flexor hallucis longus tendon transfer/augmentation. Foot Ankle Int 2000;21:1004–10.
42. Maffulli N, Leadbetter WB. Free gracilis tendon graft in neglected tears of the Achilles tendon. Clin J Sport Med 2005;15(2):56–61.
43. Kangas J, Pajala A, Ohtonen P, et al. Achilles tendon elongation after rupture repair. A randomized comparison of two postoperative regimens. Am J Sports Med 2007;35:59–64.
44. Krackow KA, Thomas SC, Jones LC. Ligament-tendon fixation: analysis of a new stitch and comparison with standard techniques. Orthopedics 1988;11:909–17.
45. Arner O, Lindholm A. Subcutaneous rupture of the Achilles tendon. A study of ninety two cases. Acta Chir Scand 1959;239:1–51.
46. Tashjian R, Hur J, Sullivan R, et al. Flexor hallucis longus transfer for repair of chronic Achilles tendinopathy. Foot Ankle Int 2003;24:673–6.
47. Mulier T, Rummens E, Dereymaeker G. Risk of neurovascular injuries in flexor hallucis longus tendon transfers: an anatomic cadaver study. Foot Ankle Int 2007;8: 910–5.
48. Dalal RB, Zenios M. The flexor hallucis longus tendon transfer for chronic tendo-achilles ruptures revisited. Ann R Coll Surg Engl 2003;85:283.
49. Frenette JP, Jackson DW. Lacerations of the flexor hallucis longus in the young athlete. J Bone Joint Surg Am 1977;59:673–6.
50. Coull R, Falvin R, Stephens MM. Flexor hallucis tendon transfer: evaluation of postoperative morbidity. Foot Ankle Int 2003;24:931–4.

51. Silver RL, de la Garza J, Rang M. The myth of muscle balance. A study of relative strengths and excursions of normal muscles about the foot and ankle. J Bone Joint Surg Br 1985;67:432–7.
52. Nellas ZJ, Loder BG, Wertheimer SJ. Reconstruction of an Achilles tendon defect utilizing an Achilles tendon allograft. J Foot Ankle Surg 1996;35:144–8 [discussion: 190].
53. Haraguchi N, Bluman E, Myerson M. Reconstruction of chronic Achilles tendon disorders with Achilles tendon allograft. Tech Foot Ankle Surg 2005;4:154–9.
54. Howard CB, Winston I, Bell W, et al. Late repair of the calcaneal tendon with carbon fibre. J Bone Joint Surg Br 1984;66:206–8.
55. Kuwada GT. Classification of tendo Achillis rupture with consideration of surgical repair techniques. J Foot Surg 1990;29:361–5.

Tendon Transfers for Achilles Reconstruction

Johnny L. Lin, MD[a,b],*

KEYWORDS

- Achilles tendinosis • Chronic Achilles rupture
- Tendon transfer

Tendon transfers are commonly used in the foot and ankle. They are used to restore function in neglected ruptures, reconstruct degenerated tendons, and correct deformity. The Achilles tendon is commonly afflicted by these problems because of the dominant role it plays in the mechanics of gait and running and its inherently poor blood supply.[1–4] Subjective symptoms are common, such as pain, swelling, diminished performance, and difficulty with shoe wear. Deformities such as a calcaneal deformity can also occur in advanced cases of Achilles deficiency, especially when they are associated with neuromuscular diseases.[5] This article is devoted to discussing the general principles of tendon transfers with regard to Achilles tendon function, the surgical techniques involved, and published results using these techniques. The goal is to provide the orthopedic foot and ankle surgeon with a wide variety of techniques to solve both the straightforward Achilles tendon problem as well as the difficult revision case.

ACHILLES TENDON PROBLEMS REQUIRING TRANSFER
Tendinosis

Tendinosis of the Achilles tendon is a common clinical problem. The mainstay of treatment has evolved around attempts at healing the tendon through rest and physical therapy.[6,7] In patients who will accept it, bracing has been used in more resistant cases. More recently, attempts at nonoperative treatment have also included the use of transdermal nitric oxide,[8,9] shockwave therapy,[10,11] and sclerotherapy.[12,13] When surgical treatment is warranted, the goals of surgery are to remove the degenerated tendon, provide a healing environment for the remaining tendon, and to restore the strength of the muscle tendon unit. Tendon transfers are added in these cases to

I have not received any funding or support in association with the content of the article I have written.

[a] Department of Orthopaedic Surgery, Rush University Medical Center, 1725 W. Harrison Street, Ste 1063, Chicago, IL 60612, USA
[b] 25 N, Winfield Road, Suite 505, Winfield, IL 60190, USA
* Corresponding author.
E-mail address: jlin@rushortho.com

provide additional collagen to the debrided tendon when an excessive amount of tendon needs to be removed.[14,15] Second, it restores lost plantar flexion strength if the gastrocsoleus complex is weakened.[14,15] Third, it improves the local blood supply when normal tendons are transferred to the area.[14–16] The generally accepted guideline for tendon transfer is when more than 50% of the tendon is abnormal[17] and the patient is older than 50.[18] Other possible indications may include poor host tissue owing to factors that are intrinsic to the patient.

Neglected Rupture

Missed ruptures of the Achilles tendon results in significant disability. Nonoperative treatment is unpredictable. The largest series of conservative treatment, 18 patients, was published in 1953. Only 56% of patients were satisfied with their treatment, which was more prolonged in nature, taking as long a several years for patients to achieve their final result.[19] Use of a solid ankle foot orthosis may also provide relief of symptoms for those who will accept the treatment. Because of these less than satisfying results, surgical treatment for neglected ruptures has gained acceptance as the optimal treatment in those who are fit to undergo surgery. The main determinant of the choice of procedure is the amount of separation between the ruptured tendon ends. When the deficiency is small, direct repair can be attempted; however, in most situations, the chronicity of the rupture results in a significant segment of tendon that requires excision, leaving a moderate gap that prevents primary apposition. In these cases, local tendinous flaps,[19–21] advancements,[22–24] autograft tissue,[25,26] or allograft tissue[27,28] can be used to restore continuity of the muscle tendinous unit. When these gaps are large or muscle degeneration has occurred within the gastrocnemius and soleus muscle, tendon transfers can provide a viable option for reconstruction. Similar to Achilles tendinosis, it provides collagen to reconstruct a "new tendon," restores lost plantar flexion strength, and improves the local blood supply. Generally accepted guidelines for tendon transfer are gaps greater than 5 cm.[17] Other possible indications may include fatty degeneration of the gastrosoleus musculature and poor host tissue owing to factors that are intrinsic to the patient.

Calcaneus Deformity

Calcaneus deformity can occur when there is an imbalance between the flexors and extensors of the ankle resulting in an increased calcaneal pitch and loss of the push-off mechanism of the foot (**Fig. 1**).[29,30] This results in a halting and thumping gait (calcaneal hitch) and sometimes a crouched gait in the setting of hamstring or psoas contractures. Symptoms include pain in the plantar heel or even ulcerations.[5] Common causes of a calcaneus deformity include myelomeningocoele[29,30] (L4 most commonly, but also L5 and sacral)[31] and poliomyelitis.[32] Tendon transfers are used in this setting to correct excessive ankle dorsiflexion and to provide a plantar flexion moment at the ankle to support the limb during the stance phase of gait. Other procedures are commonly added to the tendon tranfer(s) (ie, osteotomies and fusions) to correct associated bony deformities.

PRINCIPLES OF TENDON TRANSFERS

Tendon transfer can be an excellent tool for the foot and ankle surgeon, but it requires a keen understanding and respect of the basic principles of tendon transfers to optimize the clinical result.[33] The following concepts should be applied in the foot and ankle:

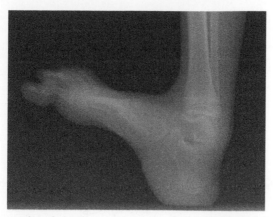

Fig. 1. Lateral radiographs of the foot and ankle with a calcaneal deformity of the foot. (*Adapted from* Park KB, Park HW, Joo SY, et al. Surgical treatment of calcaneal deformity in a select group of patients with myelomeningocele. J Bone Joint Surg Am 2008;90(10): 2149–59; with permission.)

1. Correct contractures

   Any soft tissue contracture must be corrected to provide appropriate passive range of motion. This may involve joint release or concommitant tendon lengthenings.
2. Choose the appropriate donor tendon

   The donor tendon must be of adequate strength to do the work that it is intended to do. It must contain an appropriate amount of excursion if active range of motion is to be restored. It should be relatively expendable to prevent morbidity from the transfer. It should be in phase and perform a similar duty as the replaced/reconstructed tendon to encourage neuromuscular retraining.
3. Create a straight line of pull

   Transferred tendons function best when the direction of pull is not altered. Choosing a pathway that is most direct and un-impeded will provide the most efficient function of the tendon transfer.
4. Await tissue equilibrium

   Although the need to perform tendon transfers in the face of infection or open wounds in the foot and ankle are uncommon, this situation should be avoided at all costs to prevent tendon dessication, rupture, or failure of incorporation.

PERTINENT ANATOMY

The Achilles tendon is the confluence of the medial and lateral gastrocnemius muscle and soleus muscle. It rotates 90 degrees as it inserts into the calcaneus with the fibers of the medial gastrocnemius located posteriorly.[34] At the level of the ankle, the location of the flexor and extensor tendons relative to the rotational axes of the hindfoot determines the action of each particular tendon (**Fig. 2**).[35] The relative strengths of the tendons are determined by the cross-sectional area of the muscle with the Achilles tendon having the greatest relative strength.[36] The gastrocsoleus complex (GSC) plantarflexes and inverts the foot and is by far the strongest muscle unit in the leg.

The peroneus brevis (PB) and longus (PL) tendons lie within the lateral compartment of the leg separated from the posterior compartments of the leg by the posterior intermuscular septum.[37] The two tendons insert onto the base of the fifth metatarsal and

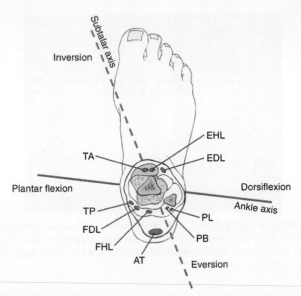

Fig. 2. The rotational axes of the ankle and subtalar joint are demonstrated. The location of each tendon with respect to these axes determines the intrinsic function of each tendon. (*Adapted from* Coughlin MJ, Schon LC. Disorders of tendons. In: Coughlin MJ, Mann RA, Saltzman CL, editors. Surgery of the Foot and Ankle. 8th edition, vol. 1. Philadelphia: Mosby Inc.; 2007. p. 1149–277; with permission.)

base of the first metatarsal respectively. At the level of the ankle they lie within the fibular groove stabilized by the superior peroneal retinaculum.[35] The PB and PL both share the roles as an evertor and plantar flexor of the ankle, whereas the PL has an additional role as a plantarflexor of the first metatarsal.[35]

The tibialis anterior (TA) tendon lies within the anterior compartment of the leg and inserts to a variable extent on the base of the first metatarsal and medial cuneiform.[37,38] It runs just underneath the superior and inferior extensor retinaculum before inserting distally. It functions as a dorsiflexor and invertor of the foot.[35]

The flexor digitorum longus (FDL) muscle originates from the posterior tibia.[37] The flexor hallucis longus (FHL) muscle originates from the posterior fibula, interosseous membrane, and adjacent intermuscular septum.[37] Both tendons travel distally through the tarsal tunnel to enter the midfoot. In the midfoot, the abductor hallucis (AH) muscle with its investing fascia conceals the deep compartment of the foot, which contains the traversing FHL and FDL. The FHL and FDL cross at the knot of Henry with the FHL passing dorsal to the FDL.[34] There are multiple interconnections between the FHL and FDL tendons within the midfoot.[39,40] This allows harvesting of the FHL or FDL proximal to the knot of Henry without losing excursion of the distal extent of the harvested tendon, but complicates harvest distal to these attachments. Distally the FHL and FDL insert on the distal phalanx of the great toe and lesser toes respectively.[37] They function mainly to flex the toes and foot, but also have a secondary function as an invertor of the foot.[35]

The tibial nerve and artery traverse the leg in the deep posterior compartment of the leg and enter into the tarsal tunnel. The tibial nerve and artery divide into the medial and lateral plantar nerve and artery and travel within the midfoot in close proximity to the FHL and FDL.[41] The neurovascular elements lie just plantar to FHL and FDL and can be at risk during tendon harvest within the midfoot.[37,40]

The medial sural nerve lies between the heads of the gastrocnemius muscle. It connects with the peroneal communicating nerve to become the sural nerve. The sural nerve runs along the midline of the calf and at a mean distance of 9.8 cm from the calcaneus, it crosses over the edge of the Achilles tendon.[42,43] It is at risk during approaches to the Achilles tendon along its course over the posterior leg and foot. After giving off the branches to the heel, the nerve runs inferior to the peroneal sheaths and can be at risk during harvesting of the peroneus brevis at its distal insertion.[43]

TYPES OF TENDON TRANSFERS
Peroneus Brevis

The use of the PB tendon has been described for use in both acute and neglected ruptures of the Achilles tendon.[14,44–46] The relative strength of the PB is over 18 times weaker than the GSC.[36] Its suitability as a donor for the Achilles tendon is supported by its being in phase with the GSC[34] during normal gait and by sharing the role as a plantarflexor of the ankle (see **Fig. 2**).[35] The tendon is in relatively close proximity to the Achilles tendon, but is contained in a separate muscle compartment.[15] Concerns with its use as a donor include loss of eversion strength and the lateral to medial pull after transfer to the calcaneus, which fails to reproduce the inversion normally created by the Achilles tendon.[15,17,47] Proponents of the technique state that the loss of eversion strength is clinically less relevant, as the peroneus longus muscle has more than twice the eversion strength of the peroneus brevis.[36] This statement is supported by the study by Gallant and colleagues[48] where eight patients had no subjective complaints despite having a statistically significant 11.9% deficit of eversion strength. The effects on the more athletic individual who may rely more heavily on the PB for ankle stabilization is unknown. Possible complications of the harvest technique include damage to the sural nerve during detachment from the base of the fifth metatarsal. This complication has not been reported or studied in detail.

PB tendon transfer to the calcaneus for Achilles tendon problems was first described by White and Kraynick[44] and popularized by Teuffer[46] for acute ruptures. The technique involved harvesting the PB tendon from its attachment at the base of the fifth metatarsal, passing it through the posterior intermuscular septum, and passing it through a transosseous drill hole in the calcaneus from lateral to medial before suturing it to the proximal stump. Thirty acute ruptures were treated with good and excellent results in all patients, with 28 of them able to return to their original level of sports activity. Turco and Spinella[14] used the PB in 40 patients, 33 of whom had acute ruptures (<1 week) and 7 of whom had neglected ruptures (1–6 weeks). Although details of the functional results were not included, the authors reported that all 40 patients returned back to sports, no morbidity from the harvest was seen, and no weakness was found. In 2001, the technique was used exclusively in neglected ruptures by Pintore and colleagues[45] They compared the results of treatment to acute ruptures with direct end-to-end anastomosis. At an average follow-up of 53 months, the patients with chronic ruptures were satisfied with the procedure, but did have a higher complication rate and greater loss of strength than the patients with acute ruptures. In conclusion, the PB is a reasonable option for treating neglected ruptures of the Achilles tendon, but concerns with weakened eversion and the need to enter a separate muscle compartment have resulted in the loss of popularity of this technique.

Surgical technique
The Achilles tendon is approached through either a medial, central, or lateral approach. After addressing the Achilles tendon pathology, the PB tendon insertion

is identified, tagged, and dissected free from the base of the fifth metatarsal. Deep dissection is then carried through the posterior incision until the posterior intermuscular septum is identified. The septum is incised and the PB tendon is brought into the posterior wound. The tendon is either anchored distally through a lateral to medial transosseus tunnel or by weaving it through the distal stump of the Achilles tendon (**Fig. 3**). The PB tendon is then brought proximally on the medial side of the Achilles tendon and sutured to the proximal stump making sure to recreate the normal resting tension of the contralateral Achilles tendon. Multiple points of fixation to the native tendon can be created with either absorbable or nonabsorbable suture.

Flexor Digitorum Longus

The use of the FDL tendon has been described for use in neglected ruptures of the Achilles tendon. The relative strength of the FDL is over 27 times weaker than the GSC.[36] Its suitability as a donor for the Achilles tendon is supported by being in phase with the GSC[34] during normal gait, by sharing the role as a plantarflexor of the ankle (see **Fig. 2**),[35] and by its relatively close proximity to the Achilles tendon. Possible concerns with its use as a donor include weakened flexion of the toes and lesser toe deformities.[47] Neither of these has been reported. Possible complications from the harvesting technique include nerve or artery injury because of the close proximity of these structures, especially when harvest is done distal to the knot of Henry. This

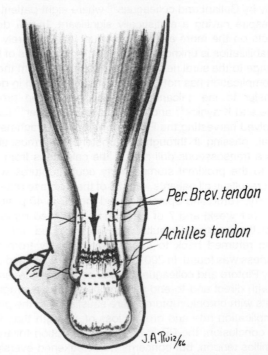

Per. Brev. tendon

Achilles tendon

J.A.Ruiz/86

Fig. 3. Peroneus brevis (PB) transfer for neglected ruptures of the Achilles tendon. After harvest of the PB tendon from the fifth metatarsal base, the posterior intermuscular septum is opened and the PB is weaved through the distal stump of the Achilles tendon. (_Reproduced from_ Turco VJ, Spinella AJ. Achilles tendon ruptures—peroneus brevis transfer. Foot Ankle 1987;7:253–9. Copyright 2009, American Orthopaedic Foot and Ankle Society Inc.; with permission. Copyright © 1987 by the American Orthopaedic Foot and Ankle Society Inc.)

has been studied in detail in cadavers[40] and although there have been several cases reported in the literature,[49] it rarely results in patient complaints.

Transfer of the FDL tendon for Achilles tendon pathology was first popularized by Mann and colleagues in 1991.[47] They studied seven patients with neglected Achilles ruptures who underwent FDL transfer at an average of 39 months postop and had six excellent/good results and one fair result. No re-ruptures were seen. A more recent study by Qu and colleagues[49] retrospectively reviewed five patients who had an FDL transfer for chronic Achilles rupture at an average follow-up of 24 months and found excellent results in one case, good results in three cases, and a poor result in one case. In conclusion, although good results have been obtained with the FDL transfer, it requires dissection around the neurovascular bundle and is weaker and farther from the Achilles tendon than the FHL.[15] As a result, most surgeons prefer using the FHL tendon for Achilles tendon pathology. Nevertheless, the FDL transfer remains a viable option with minimal morbidity in patients who are not candidates for a FHL transfer.

Surgical technique

The Achilles tendon is approached through either a medial, central, or lateral approach. After addressing the Achilles tendon pathology, the FDL tendon is harvested from the midfoot. The incision is made over the medial midfoot, just above the dorsal edge of the AH muscle from the navicular to the neck of the first metatarsal. The AH and the flexor digitorum brevis muscles are dissected free from the first metatarsal and retracted plantarly to expose the contents of the midfoot. The FHL and FDL are identified in the proximal end of the wound and dissected distally. If a longer graft is needed, the knot of Henry is released and the dissection is carried distal taking care to identify and divide the interconnections between the FHL and FDL. Special attention should be paid to protecting the neurovascular elements as they are at greatest risk at and distal to the knot of Henry. After an appropriate graft length is exposed, the FDL is tenodesed to the FHL with the toes and ankle in a neutral position using nonabsorbable suture (**Fig. 4**A). The FDL is then tenotomized, tagged, and brought into the proximal wound posterior to the neurovascular bundle. A transosseus tunnel is created in the calcaneus and the tendon is brought from medial to lateral through the tunnel before anastamosing the FDL with the Achilles tendon by either weaving the FDL through the Achilles or using side-to-side approximation with nonabsorbable suture (**Fig. 4**B). Alternatively, suture anchors or an interference screw can be used to anchor the tendon distally. Regardless of technique, care is taken to re-create the normal resting tension of the contralateral ankle.

Flexor Hallucis Longus

The use of the FHL tendon has been described for use in Achilles tendinosis and chronic Achilles ruptures. The relative strength of the FHL is more than 13 times weaker than the GSC despite being the second strongest plantarflexor of the ankle.[36] Its suitability as a donor for the Achilles tendon is supported by being in phase with the GSC[34] during normal gait, sharing the role as a plantar flexor of the ankle (see **Fig. 2**)[35] and being in the closest proximity to the Achilles tendon.[15] The distally situated muscle belly also theoretically provides a more vascular environment to improve healing in the region.[15,16,50] Concerns with its use as a donor include loss of push-off strength during gait, resultant clawed hallux deformity, and transfer metatarsalgia.[51,52] Coull and colleagues[52] studied the morbidity following FHL transfer for Achilles tendinosis and chronic Achilles ruptures and found that despite loss of active interphalangeal joint flexion, there were insignificant changes in pedobarographic pressures, an

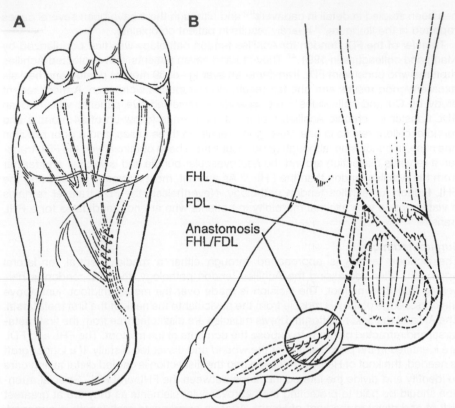

Fig. 4. Flexor digitorum longus (FDL) transfer for Achilles tendinosis. Harvest of the FDL is shown in the midfoot with tenodesis of the distal end of the FDL with the flexor hallucis longus (A). The FDL is then anchored distally through a drill hole in the calcaneus and sutured back on itself (B). (*Adapted from* Mann RA, Holmes GB Jr., Seale KS, et al. Chronic rupture of the Achilles tendon: a new technique of repair. J Bone Joint Surg Am 1991;73: 214–9; with permission.)

average American Orthopaedic Foot and Ankle Society (AOFAS) Hallux score of 97, and no impairment in walking, running, stair climbing, or rising from a crouched position because of weakness of the great toe. Further support for the FHL tendon as a donor can be extrapolated from the report of benign neglect in four athletes with FHL tendon lacerations that resulted in no apparent disability.[53] Despite the overwhelming approval the FHL as a donor tendon, there has been a case report of a flexible cock-up toe deformity has been reported after FHL transfer where the distal limb of the FHL was not tenodesed with the FDL.[51] No other cases have been reported. Possible complications from the harvesting technique are identical to those for the FDL, which include nerve or artery injury, especially when the harvest is done distal to the knot of Henry.[40] In cadaver specimens, up to 33% of specimens had either a stretching, partial rupture, or complete rupture of either the medial or lateral plantar nerve.[40] Clinically apparent symptoms have rarely been reported.[54] Attempts to limit this morbidity led to a single-incision technique where the FHL is harvested through the original posterior hindfoot.[50] This results in a graft that is an average of 3 cm shorter compared with harvesting in the midfoot.[55] Interference screws and suture anchors have been added to the technique to overcome these shorter graft lengths.[56]

FHL tendon transfer to the calcaneus for Achilles tendon problems was first described by Hansen in 1991 for neglected ruptures.[57] Clinical results were first published by Wapner and colleagues[15] in 1993 on seven patients with chronic Achilles ruptures. The technique involved harvesting the FHL from the midfoot and transferring the tendon through a transosseous drill hole in the calcaneus and weaving it through the Achilles tendon (**Fig. 5**). Six of seven patients had a good or excellent result, whereas one patient had a fair result. Instrumented strength testing revealed a 29.5% loss of plantarflexion power. There were no re-ruptures and patients returned to their preoperative recreational activities. In a more recent series, Elias and colleagues[56] studied 15 patients with neglected ruptures with 5-cm or larger gaps using a single-incision technique with an associated V-Y lengthening. At an average of 2 years follow-up the average AOFAS score was 94.1 with all patients satisfied with their outcome. Instrumented strength testing revealed a 22.3% loss of strength. There were no forefoot complaints despite the patients' perception of less strength with great toe. Multiple authors have also reported on the use of the FHL transfer to treat both insertional and noninsertional Achilles tendinopathy.[16,50,58,59] Den Hartog[50] reported on the treatment of 27 patients with insertional Achilles tendinopathy with debridement, bone resection, and FHL transfer. He used the one-incision technique to reduce the morbidity of the procedure. At a mean follow-up of 35 months, the AO-FAS scores improved from 41.7 to 90.1. There were no hyperextension deformities of the hallux or hammertoe deformities at final follow-up. Martin and colleagues[58] studied 44 patients with noninsertional Achilles tendinopathy who had debridement and FHL transfer using the two-incision technique. At a mean follow-up of 3.4 years, the average AOFAS score was 91.7. Instrumented strength deficits averaged 30% less than the contralateral limb; 95.5% of patients had improvements in pain and

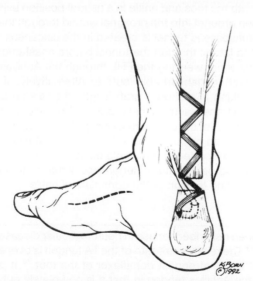

Fig. 5. Flexor hallucis longus (FHL) transfer for Achilles tendinosis using the two-incision technique. After harvest from the midfoot, the FHL tendon is anchored distally through a drill hole in the calcaneus and weaved through the distal and proximal tendon stumps. (*Reproduced from* Wapner KL, Hecht PJ, Shea JR, et al. Anatomy of second muscular layer of the foot: considerations for tendon selection in transfer for Achilles and posterior tibial tendon reconstruction. Foot Ankle Int 1994;15(8):420–3, Copyright © 1994 by the American Orthopaedic Foot and Ankle Society Inc.)

86.4% were satisfied with the result. No ruptures or forefoot complaints were reported. In addition to clinical results, Hahn and colleagues[16] looked at the MRI findings at 3.8 years follow-up in 13 patients after FHL transfer and showed that none of the cases had signs of inflammation or hypervascularity. Six had a homogeneous tendon mass, five had a thin layer of interposed tissue between the FHL and Achilles tendon, and in only one could the original weaving of the FHL tendon through the Achilles tendon be seen. They concluded that there is excellent tendon incorporation after tendon transfer. Furthermore, the volume of the muscle belly of the FHL tendon showed an average increase of 17%, showing continued function and adaptation to its new role. In conclusion, the FHL transfer is the preferred technique for reconstruction of Achilles tendinosis or neglected ruptures because of its superior donor characteristics, good clinical results, and MRI-proven incorporation into the native tendon.

Surgical technique

The Achilles tendon is approached through a medial, central, or lateral approach. After addressing the Achilles tendon pathology, the FHL tendon is harvested either through the posterior incision (single incision technique) or from the midfoot (two-incision technique). In the single-incision technique, the dissection is carried anteriorly until the posterior fascia of the leg is encountered. The fascia is then divided longitudinally making sure to release proximally enough to allow free movement of the FHL muscle belly. The identity of the FHL tendon is verified by noting flexion of the hallux with traction on the tendon. The neurovascular bundle is then gently retracted medially and with the foot and hallux maximally plantarflexed, the tendon is tenotomized as distal as possible from medial to lateral. If a two-incision technique is used, a second incision is made over the medial foot using the identical technique for harvesting the FDL as outlined previously. After an appropriate graft length is exposed, the FHL is tenodesed to the FDL with the toes and ankle in a neutral position using nonabsorbable suture. The FHL is then brought into the proximal wound through the incised posterior fascia of the leg. A transosseus tunnel is created in the calcaneus and the tendon is brought from medial to lateral through the tunnel before anastamosing the FHL with the Achilles tendon by either weaving the FHL through the Achilles or using side-to-side approximation with nonabsorbable suture. Alternatively, if a single-incision technique is used resulting in a shorter graft length, the tendon can be fixed using an interference screw. A transosseus tunnel is created from just anterior to the Achilles tendon to the plantar aspect of the calcaneus. Using a beath pin, the FHL is then pulled into the tunnel and tensioned by pulling the sutures through the bottom of the foot. An interference screw is then inserted and multiple points of fixation to the native tendon are created using nonabsorbable suture. Regardless of the technique, care is taken to re-create the normal resting tension of the contralateral ankle.

Tibialis Anterior

The TA tendon has been described for use in neuromuscular diseases for a nonspastic deficient GSC.[31,60–63] The relative strength of the TA tendon is over eight times weaker than the GSC, but it is the strongest dorsiflexor of the foot.[36] It is poorly suited as a primary donor for the Achilles tendon in that it is completely out of phase with the GSC.[34] During normal gait, its role as a dorsiflexor is antagonistic to the GSC (see **Fig. 2**),[35] and it is located a long distance from the Achilles tendon. Despite being a poor candidate to replace the function of the GSC, its function as a tendon transfer in this situation is to correct a muscle imbalance where all or most of the muscles of the posterior compartment are deficient, leaving no better option. Concerns with its use as a donor include overcorrection and resultant equinus deformity.[31,60–63] Although it is beyond the scope of this article, additional procedures such as osteotomies, fusions, tendon releases, and concommitant tendon transfers should be chosen on a case-by-case basis to fully correct the underlying boney and dynamic deformity.

The results of TA transfer for paralytic disorders of the foot was first described by Peabody in 1938 to treat paralytic disease caused by poliomyelitis.[64] Because of worldwide vaccination against the disease, there are no recent reports of TA transfer for calcaneal deformities attributable to polio. One of the larger reports in the literature

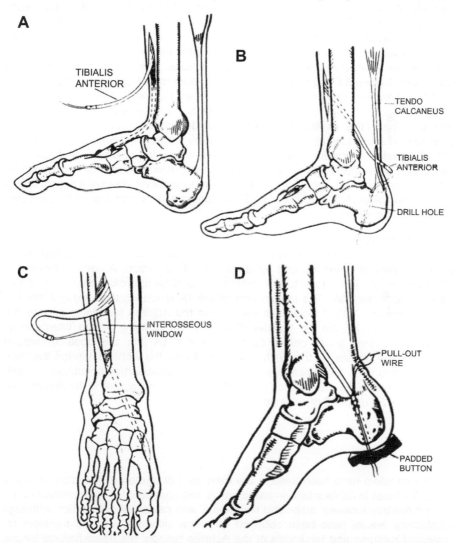

Fig. 6. Anterior tibial (AT) transfer through the interosseous membrane for calcaneal deformity of the ankle. The AT tendon is detached from its insertion and tagged (*A*). A posterior incision is created to identify the insertion site just anterior to the Achilles tendon (*B*). A third incision is created over the anterior leg and the AT tendon is passed proximally to this incision. An opening in the interosseous membrane is created (*C*), the tendon is passed into the posterior incision and anchored through a drill hole in the calcaneus (*D*). (*Adapted from* Georgiadis GM, Aronson DD. Posterior transfer of the anterior tibial tendon in children who have a myelomeningocele. J Bone Joint Surg Am 1990;72(3):392–8; with permission.)

was in 1956 by Herndon and colleagues[32] who reported on the results of 12 patients at an average of 3 years follow-up. He obtained good and excellent results in 10 of the 12 patients. Reports of TA transfer for the treatment of myelomeningocoele have been more numerous. Bliss and Menelaus[65] studied the long-term results of 46 feet in 25 patients at a minimum of 12 years follow-up. Mild residual calcaneal deformity or secondary equinus deformity was found in 25 of 46 feet and only 10 feet did not require subsequent surgery after the TA tendon transfer. Despite this, they recommended TA transfer to limit the progression of deformity. More optimistic results were obtained by Georgiadis and Aronson[62] when they reviewed 39 feet in 20 patients at an average of 6 years follow-up and found that satisfactory results were obtained in 95% of feet. However, up to 26% needed subsequent soft tissue and osseous procedures for secondary deformities. They noted that those with lower-level disease (L5 and sacral) and patients older than 4 did best. These findings were supported by Fraser and Hoffman[65] when they studied 46 feet in 26 patients at 8.4 years follow-up and found that the satisfaction rate was 89%. However, they observed that 76% of feet had secondary deformities. They also found that lower-level disease (sacral) responded best to the surgery. In conclusion, it appears that TA transfer is a useful operation to prevent worsening of a calcaneal deformity with a high satisfaction rate in the setting of myelomeningocoele and poliomyelitis. In myelomeningocoele, the best results were in lower-level disease (L5 and sacral) and in those older than 4. Secondary deformities are likely and should be expected and treated accordingly.

Surgical technique
An incision is made over the TA tendon insertion over the base of the first metatarsal and medial cuneiform and released from its insertion. A second incision is made proximally, just lateral to the anterior tibial crest approximately 6 cm above the ankle joint (**Fig. 6**A). The tagged end of the TA tendon is then brought into the proximal wound. A third incision is made over the Achilles tendon to expose the site of insertion for the TA transfer (**Fig. 6**B). An opening in the interosseous membrane is then made before passage of the TA into the posterior wound (**Fig. 6**C). The transfer is then either anchored into the Achilles tendon insertion and periosteum of the calcaneus with multiple nonabsorbable sutures or with suture anchors or an interference screw (**Fig. 6**D). The transfer is tensioned with the ankle in 20 degrees of equinus.

SUMMARY

Tendon transfers have been used in the treatment of tendon dysfunction for many years. Their use in Achilles tendon pathology is well accepted for the treatment of neglected Achilles ruptures, advanced tendinosis, and calcaneal deformities. Although satisfactory results have been obtained for many different types of transfers for neglected ruptures and tendinosis of the Achilles tendon, the flexor hallucis longus tendon has gained the most approval because of its superior donor characteristics and good clinical results. In calcaneal deformities secondary to poliomyelitis and myelomeningocoele, the use of the tibialis anterior tendon transfer remains one of the cornerstones of a reconstructive procedure to prevent progression of deformity and improve quality of life. By understanding the basic principles of tendon transfers and choosing the appropriate donor, these difficult clinical problems can be treated with the optimal technique to ensure the best possible result.

REFERENCES

1. Lagergen C, Lindoholm A. Vascular distribution in Achilles tendon— an angiographic study. Acta Chir Scand 1958;116:491–5.
2. Zantop T, Tillmann B, Petersen W. Quantitative assessment of blood vessels of the human Achilles tendon: an immunohistochemical cadaver study. Arch Orthop Trauma Surg 2003;123(9):501–4.
3. Ahmed IM, Lagopoulos M, McConnell P, et al. Blood supply of the Achilles tendon. J Orthop Res 1998;16(5):591–6.
4. Astrom M, Westin N. Blood flow in the human Achilles tendon assessed by laser Doppler flowmetry. J Orthop Res 1994;12(2):246–52.
5. Dhillon MS, Sandhu HS. Surgical options in the management of residual foot problems in poliomyelitis. Foot Ankle Clin 2000;5(2):327–47.
6. Ohberg L, Lorentzon R, Alfredson H. Good clinical results but persisting side-to-side differences in calf muscle strength after surgical treatment of chronic Achilles tendinosis: a 5-year follow-up. Scand J Med Sci Sports 2001;11(4):207–12.
7. Angermann P, Hovgaard D. Chronic Achilles tendinopathy in athletic individuals: results of nonsurgical treatment. Foot Ankle Int 1999;20(5):304–6.
8. Paoloni JA, Appleyard RC, Nelson J, et al. Topical glyceryl trinitrate treatment of chronic noninsertional achilles tendinopathy. A randomized, double-blind, placebo-controlled trial. J Bone Joint Surg Am 2004;86(5):916–22.
9. Paoloni JA, Murrell GA. Three-year follow up study of topical glyceryl trinitrate treatment of chronic noninsertional Achilles tendinopathy. Foot Ankle Int 2007;28(10):1064–8.
10. Costa ML, Shepstone L, Donell ST, et al. Shock wave therapy for chronic Achilles tendon pain: a randomized placebo-controlled trial. Clin Orthop Relat Res 2005;440:199–204.
11. Rompe JD. Shock wave therapy for chronic Achilles tendon pain: a randomized placebo-controlled trial. Clin Orthop Relat Res 2006;445:276–7.
12. Boesen MI, Torp-Pedersen S, Koenig MJ, et al. Ultrasound guided electrocoagulation in patients with chronic non-insertional Achilles tendinopathy: a pilot study. Br J Sports Med 2006;40(9):761–6.
13. Alfredson H, Ohberg L. Increased intratendinous vascularity in the early period after sclerosing injection treatment in Achilles tendinosis: a healing response? Knee Surg Sports Traumatol Arthrosc 2006;14(4):399–401.
14. Turco VJ, Spinella AJ. Achilles tendon ruptures—peroneus brevis transfer. Foot Ankle 1987;7:253–9.
15. Wapner KL, Pavlock GS, Hecht PJ, et al. Repair of chronic Achilles tendon rupture with flexor hallucis longus tendon transfer. Foot Ankle 1993;14:443–9.
16. Hahn F, Meyer P, Maiwald C, et al. Treatment of chronic Achilles tendinopathy and ruptures with flexor hallucis tendon transfer: clinical outcome and MRI findings. Foot Ankle Int 2008;29(8):794–802.
17. Myerson MS. Achilles tendon ruptures. Instr Course Lect 1999;48:219–30.
18. McGarvey WC, Palumbo RC, Baxter DE, et al. Insertional Achilles tendinosis: surgical treatment through a central tendon splitting approach. Foot Ankle Int 2002;23(1):19–25.
19. Christensen I. Rupture of the Achilles tendon: analysis of 57 cases. Acta Chir Scand 1953;106:50–60.
20. Arner O, Lindholm A, Orell SR. Histologic changes in subcutaneous rupture of the Achilles tendon; a study of 74 cases. Acta Chir Scand 1959;116:484–90.

21. Us AK, Bilgin SS, Aydin T, et al. Repair of neglected Achilles tendon ruptures: procedures and functional results. Arch Orthop Trauma Surg 1997;116: 408–11.

22. Abraham E, Pankovich AM. Neglected rupture of the Achilles tendon. Treatment by V-Y tendinous flap. J Bone Joint Surg Am 1975;57:253–5.

23. Leitner A, Voigt C, Rahmanzadeh R. Treatment of extensive aseptic defects in old Achilles tendon ruptures: methods and case reports. Foot Ankle 1992;13:176–80.

24. Parker RG, Repinecz M. Neglected rupture of the achilles tendon. Treatment by modified Strayer gastrocnemius recession. J Am Podiatry Assoc 1979;69:548–55.

25. Zadek I. Repair of old rupture of the tendo Achillis by means of fascia lata: report of a case. J Bone Joint Surg Am 1940;22:1070–1.

26. Bugg El Jr, Boyd BM. Repair of neglected rupture or laceration of the Achilles tendon. Clin Orthop Relat Res 1968;6:73–5.

27. Nellas ZJ, Loder BG, Wertheimer SJ. Reconstruction of an Achilles tendon defect utilizing an Achilles tendon allograft. J Foot Ankle Surg. 1996;35:144–8, 190.

28. Haraguchi N, Bluman EM, Myerson MS. Reconstruction of chronic Achilles tendon disorders with Achilles tendon allograft. Special focus. Tech Foot Ankle Surg. 2005;4:154–9.

29. Broughton NS, Menelaus MB. The orthopaedic management of myelodysplasia and spina bifida. In: Chapman MW, editor. Chapman's orthopaedic surgery. 3rd edition. Philadelphia: Lippincott Williams and Wilkins; 2001. p. 4567.

30. Noonan KJ. Myelomeningocele: calcaneal deformity. In: Morrissy RT, Weinstein SL, editors, Lovell and Winter's pediatric orthopaedics. 6th edition, vol. 1. Philadelphia: Lippincott Williams and Wilkins; 2006. p. 631.

31. Park KB, Park HW, Joo SY, et al. Surgical treatment of calcaneal deformity in a select group of patients with myelomeningocele. J Bone Joint Surg Am 2008; 90(10):2149–59.

32. Herndon CH, Stron JM, Heyman CH. Transposition of the tibialis anterior in the treatment of paralytic talipes calcaneus. J Bone Joint Surg Am 1956;38:751–60.

33. Green DP. Radial nerve palsy. In: Green DP, Hotchkiss RN, Pederson WC, editors, Green's operative hand surgery. 4th edition, vol. 2. New York: Churchill Livingstone; 1999. p. 1481–96.

34. Sarrafian SK. Functional anatomy of the foot and ankle. In: Sarrafian Shahan K, editor. Anatomy of the foot and ankle. 2nd edition. Philadelphia: J.B. Lippincott Company; 1993. p. 474–602.

35. Coughlin MJ, Schon LC. Disorders of tendons. In: Coughlin MJ, Mann RA, Saltzman CL, editors, Surgery of the foot and ankle. 8th edition, vol. 1. Philadelphia: Mosby Inc; 2007. p. 1149–277.

36. Silver RL, de la Garza J, Rang M. The myth of muscle balance. A study of relative strengths and excursions of normal muscles about the foot and ankle. J Bone Joint Surg Br 1985;67:432–7.

37. Netter FH. Atlas of human anatomy. 2nd edition. East Hanover (NJ): Novartis Pharmaceuticals Corporation; 1999. p. 481–506.

38. Anagnostakos K, Bachelier F, Fürst OA, et al. Rupture of the anterior tibial tendon: three clinical cases, anatomical study, and literature review. Foot Ankle Int 2006; 27(5):330–9.

39. Wapner KL, Hecht PJ, Shea JR, et al. Anatomy of second muscular layer of the foot: considerations for tendon selection in transfer for Achilles and posterior tibial tendon reconstruction. Foot Ankle Int 1994;15(8):420–3.

40. Mulier T, Rummens E, Dereymaeker G. Risk of neurovascular injuries in flexor hallucis longus tendon transfers: an anatomic cadaver study. Foot Ankle Int 2007; 28(8):910–5.
41. Havel PE, Ebraheim NA, Clark SE, et al. Tibial branching in the tarsal tunnel. Foot Ankle 1988;9:117–9.
42. Webb J, Moorjani N, Radford M. Anatomy of the sural nerve and its relation to the Achilles tendon. Foot Ankle Int 2000;21(6):475–7.
43. Aktan Ikiz ZA, Uçerler H, Bilge O. The anatomic features of the sural nerve with an emphasis on its clinical importance. Foot Ankle Int 2005;26(7):560–7.
44. White RK, Kraynick BM. Surgical uses of the peroneus brevis tendon. Surg Gynecol Obstet 1959;108:117–21.
45. Pintore E, Barra V, Pintore R, et al. Peroneus brevis tendon transfer in neglected tears of the Achilles tendon. J Trauma 2001;50:71–8.
46. Teuffer AP. Traumatic rupture of the Achilles tendon. Reconstruction by transplant and graft using the lateral peroneus brevis. Orthop Clin North Am 1974; 5:89–93.
47. Mann RA, Holmes GB Jr, Seale KS, et al. Chronic rupture of the Achilles tendon: a new technique of repair. J Bone Joint Surg Am 1991;73:214–9.
48. Gallant GG, Massie C, Turco VJ. Assessment of eversion and plantar flexion strength after repair of Achilles tendon rupture using peroneus brevis tendon transfer. Am J Orthop 1995;24(3):257–61.
49. Qu JF, Cao LH, Zhao HB, et al. [Flexor digitorum (hallucis) longus muscle tendon transfer in the repair of old rupture of the Achilles tendon] Zhongguo Gu Shang 2008;21(4):297–9 [in Chinese].
50. Den Hartog BD. Flexor hallucis longus transfer for chronic Achilles tendonosis. Foot Ankle Int 2003;24(3):233–7.
51. Herbst SA, Miller SD. Transection of the medial plantar nerve and hallux cock-up deformity after flexor hallucis longus tendon transfer for Achilles tendinitis: case report. Foot Ankle Int 2006;27(8):639–41.
52. Coull R, Flavin R, Stephens MM. Flexor hallucis longus tendon transfer: evaluation of postoperative morbidity. Foot Ankle Int 2003;24(12):931–4.
53. Frenette JP, Jackson DW. Lacerations of the flexor hallucis longus in the young athlete. J Bone Joint Surg Am 1977;59:673–6.
54. Myerson MS, Corrigan J. Medial plantar nerve paresthesias: treatment of posterior tibial tendon dysfunction with flexor digitorum longus tendon transfer and calcaneal osteotomy. Orthopedics 1996;19:383–8.
55. Tashjian RZ, Hur J, Sullivan RJ, et al. Flexor hallucis longus transfer for repair of chronic Achilles tendinopathy. Foot Ankle Int 2003;24:673–6.
56. Elias I, Besser M, Nazarian LN, et al. Reconstruction for missed or neglected Achilles tendon rupture with V-Y lengthening and flexor hallucis longus tendon transfer through one incision. Foot Ankle Int 2007;28(12):1238–48.
57. Hansen ST. Trauma to the heel cord. In: Jahss MH, editor, Disorders of the foot and ankle, vol. 3. Philadelphia: W.B. Saunders; 1991. p. 2355–60.
58. Martin RL, Manning CM, Carcia CR, et al. An outcome study of chronic Achilles tendinosis after excision of the Achilles tendon and flexor hallucis longus tendon transfer. Foot Ankle Int 2005;26(9):691–7.
59. Wilcox DK, Bohay DR, Anderson JG. Treatment of chronic achilles tendon disorders with flexor hallucis longus tendon transfer/augmentation. Foot Ankle Int 2000;21(12):1004–10.

60. Fernández-Feliberti R, Fernández SA, Colón C, et al. Transfer of the tibialis anterior for calcaneus deformity in myelodysplasia. J Bone Joint Surg Am 1992;74(7): 1038–41.
61. Fraser RK, Hoffman EB. Calcaneus deformity in the ambulant patient with myelomeningocele. J Bone Joint Surg Br 1991;73(6):994–7.
62. Georgiadis GM, Aronson DD. Posterior transfer of the anterior tibial tendon in children who have a myelomeningocele. J Bone Joint Surg Am 1990;72(3):392–8.
63. Turner JW, Cooper RR. Posterior transposition of tibialis anterior through the interosseous membrane. Clin Orthop Relat Res 1971;79:71–4.
64. Peabody C. Tendon transposition in the paralytic foot. In: American Academy of Orthopedic Surgeons: instructional course lectures, vol. 6. Ann Arbor: J W Edwards; 1949. p. 178–88.
65. Bliss DG, Menelaus MB. The results of transfer of the tibialis anterior to the heel in patients who have a myelomeningocele. J Bone Joint Surg Am 1986;68(8): 1258–64.

Complications of the Treatment of Achilles Tendon Ruptures

Andy Molloy, FRCS (Tr & Orth)[a],*, Edward V. Wood, FRCS (Tr & Orth)[b]

KEYWORDS

• Achilles • Tendon • Treatment • Complications • Rupture

The first complication of the Achilles tendon was recorded in Greek mythology as the weakened area or vulnerability that would ultimately deliver death to the god, Achilles, himself. Achilles was invulnerable to mortal blows, having been dipped as an infant in the River Styx by his mother Thetis. However, the heel she held him by, which was therefore penetrable, was to be his undoing. With pinpoint accuracy, a poisoned shaft, loosened from Paris' bow, struck his heel, mortally wounding him.[1]

The Achilles tendon is the confluence of the gastrocnemius and soleus muscles. It is the largest and strongest tendon in the body, having to withstand up to eight times body weight in force when undertaking sporting activities. Since first described by Hippocrates in ancient times and Ambroise Pare in modern times, treatment of the Achilles tendon, and especially its rupture, has been fraught with complications.[2,3] With the advent of modern techniques, the rates of complications have diminished; however, when they occur, they still bring significant morbidity and are technically challenging to treat. This article delineates the complications of treatment of the Achilles tendon, their incidence and treatment, and methods for their potential avoidance.

RERUPTURE
Introduction

Polaillon performed the first reported repair of an acute Achilles tendon rupture in 1888, with the first major study comparing operative and nonoperative repair of these ruptures being reported by Qenu and Stoianovitch in 1929.[4] Ever since that time, controversy has raged as to the potential risks and benefits of both modes of treatment. The major reasons for such interest in operative management of Achilles tendon ruptures have been the functional results and especially the rate of rerupture following nonoperative treatment. Reruptures of the Achilles tendon occur for several reasons, the first being decreased mechanical strength of the fibrous scar tissue as compared

[a] University Hospital Aintree, Longmoor Lane, Liverpool L9 7AL, UK
[b] Countess of Chester Hospital, Liverpool Road, Chester, Cheshire CH2 1UL, UK
* Corresponding author.
E-mail address: orthoblue@aol.com (A. Molloy).

Foot Ankle Clin N Am 14 (2009) 745–759
doi:10.1016/j.fcl.2009.07.004
1083-7515/09/$ – see front matter © 2009 Elsevier Inc. All rights reserved.

foot.theclinics.com

with that of normal tendon. Failure of this scar tissue may occur in two scenarios. The first is of a single insult to the healed Achilles tendon, in which the force of this insult exceeds the yield point of the tissue (ie, after return to sporting activities after injury). The second scenario is where repeated low-level stressing of the healed tendon in activities of daily living causes failure of the scar tissue. This scenario is more common with a background of the second reason for a predilection to rerupture, a pathologic process causing abnormal morphology of the Achilles tendon before the index injury. Pajala and colleagues[5] found that there was a higher incidence of complications of treatment of the index Achilles rupture in those who had sustained the rupture during low-energy activities of daily living. It is presumed that the rupture was secondary to a tendinopathic process, either with or without symptoms, together with the patient' systemic factors such as smoking, diabetes, and corticosteroid usage.

Incidence

Bhandari and colleagues[6] published a meta-analysis of treatment of acute Achilles tendon ruptures in 2002. They identified 273 citations, of which only six studies were eligible for inclusion in the meta-analysis due to scientific robustness. The studies' pooled data showed that surgical repair significantly reduced the risk of rerupture as compared with conservative treatment. The respective rates were 3.1% and 13%. They hypothesized that these results demonstrated that for every 10 patients treated operatively, one rerupture could be prevented as compared with if the patients had been treated nonoperatively.

Khan and colleagues[7] published their meta-analysis in 2005. They, however, looked at all randomized controlled trials comparing operative and nonoperative treatment and the effect of different mobilization regimes. They identified 36 trials, of which only 12 were suitable for inclusion because of the stringent inclusion criteria. They discounted three of the studies included in the meta-analysis by Bhandari and colleagues because of inadequate reporting of results, discontinuation of treatment in the control group, and inadequate randomization. Kahn and colleagues' meta-analysis of pooled data demonstrated rerupture rates of 3.5% in the operatively treated group and 12.6% in the nonoperative group. This correlated to a relative risk of 0.27. The mean duration of follow-up ranged from 8 to 30 months. Two studies were included for the comparison of open and percutaneous operative repair. Lim and colleagues[8] found no significant difference between the two groups. The pooled data found rerupture rates of 4.3% in the open group and 2.1% in the percutaneous group. There has been one further significant prospective randomized study published since the aforementioned meta-analysis by Wagnon and Akayi.[9] Their study compared open repair with the Webb-Bannister technique.[10] They reported a rerupture rate of 5.7% in the open group and 4.5% in the percutaneous group from their cohort of 57 patients.

There is a paucity of specific treatment of reruptures of the Achilles tendon. Pajala and colleagues[5] reported an increase in the annual incidence of acute Achilles tendon rupture in their hospital's catchment area and a concomitant rise in the rerupture rate (from 0.25 per 100,000 from 1979 to 1990 to 3.5 per 100,000 in 1999). This represented a rerupture rate of 5.6% in the 409 patients they retrospectively reviewed. The rerupture was treated nonoperatively in 4 patients and operatively in 19 patients. The operative repair also was treated by augmentation in 15 out of the 19 patients; these included gastrocnemius fascial turndowns, turndown flaps, plantaris tendons, and one case of augmentation with exogenous material. There were two further reruptures following the secondary operative procedure. The mean isokinetic peak torque deficit was 10.3%, and the mean isometric strength deficit was 14.4%. Six patients were completely pain-free; five were mildly painful, and one patient had moderate pain. Four patients reported moderate subjective stiffness, with only one having objective restriction of range of movement. Only one patient was satisfied with major reservations, the others being very satisfied or satisfied with minor reservations.

Treatment

Although reruptures of the Achilles tendon may be purely acute (ie, forceful trauma through a well-healed tendon) and resemble an acute primary rupture, they are frequently acute on chronic. By this, it is meant that gradual failure has begun to occur over a period of time, with a final episode in which there has been complete failure of the fibrous tissue from the healing of the primary rupture. This is often with minimal trauma. The typical appearance is of a chronically inflamed swollen Achilles with an indiscrete palpable gap, a resting habitus of increased dorsiflexion, and an abnormal Simmonds test (**Fig. 1**). The authors always obtain a magnetic resonance imaging (MRI) scan as part of preoperative work-up. In addition to delineating the length of the tendon defect, it provides useful information on the morphology of the tendon ends and any pathologic processes contributing to this morphology.

In the authors' practice, the operation is performed under general anesthetic with the patient prone. A thigh tourniquet is used, as a calf tourniquet will alter the tension from the proximal muscle mass. It is essential that both legs are prepared and draped, so that accurate estimation of tendon tension can be made from the degree of resting plantarflexion of the feet (**Fig. 2**). A standard approach is made over the tendon rerupture site, with careful dissection so as not to unduly traumatize the soft tissues. Self-retainers are not used, and attempts are made to only retract on one side of the incision at a time. The fibrous tissue at the rerupture site, which frequently is elongated and in partial continuity, is excised (**Fig. 3**). The tendon ends then are debrided back to healthy tissue (**Fig. 4**). If extensive and severe tendinopathy is present upon preoperative MRI, an on-table decision will have to be made between compromising the tendon debridement and augmenting the repair, or a thorough debridement with

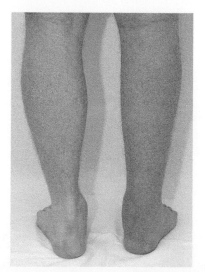

Fig. 1. Clinical photograph of patient with rerupture of right Achilles tendon.

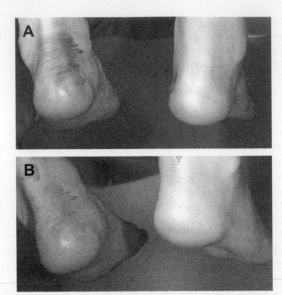

Fig. 2. Clinical photograph of patient lying prone on operating table with rerupture of the Achilles tendon. (*A*) Before repair. (*B*) After repair.

more substantial augmentation techniques. These augmentation techniques are the same as those described for chronic Achilles tendon ruptures.[11]

If the postdebridement defect is around 2.5 cm or less, then a direct end-to-end repair is performed with minimal mobilization of the tendon ends. If this places the foot into undue plantarflexion (as compared with the contralateral leg) or if the defect is up to around 4.5 cm, then the approach is extended, and a proximal V-Y advancement is performed. A direct end-to-end repair then may be performed (**Fig. 5**).

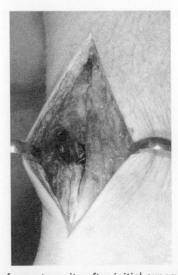

Fig. 3. Clinical photograph of rerupture site after initial exposure.

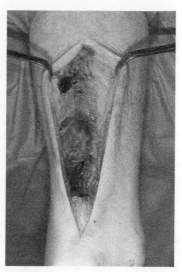

Fig. 4. Clinical photograph of rerupture site after debridement.

It is necessary to carefully repair the paratenon so as to minimize the chances of adhesions. There then should be a careful apposition of the superficial soft tissues followed by skin closure. This is performed with interrupted nonabsorbable sutures as, in the authors' experience, minor wound problems and stitch abscesses may occur when absorbable sutures are not absorbed wholly in this relatively hypovascular area.

SURAL NERVE MORBIDITY
Introduction

The incidence of sural nerve damage following treatment varies according to the technique used and between series using the same technique. In a quantitative review, Lo

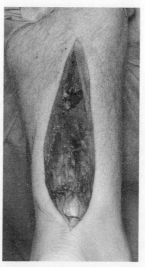

Fig. 5. Clinical photograph after repair of rerupture.

and colleagues[12] found an overall rate of 6.0% (N=42) sural nerve damage in 701 operatively treated cases.

Anatomy

In most cases, the sural nerve forms from the medial sural cutaneous nerve and the peroneal communicating branch of the lateral sural cutaneous nerve.[13] These join in the midline 11 to 20 cm proximal to the lateral malleolus and run distally to a point approximately 17.5 mm from the lateral border of the tendo-Achilles at its insertion in the os calcis, before passing into the foot.[13] It crosses the lateral border of the tendoachilles (TA) at a mean of 9.8 cm from its insertion.[13] There is, however, considerable variation, such that even distally the nerve may only be 3 mm from the lateral border of the TA.[13] Webb concluded that because of this variation, percutaneous sutures should not be placed in the lateral half of the TA.[13]

This view is supported further by a cadaveric, biomechanical, comparison of open and percutaneous TA repair following a simulated rupture undertaken by Hockenbury and Johns.[14] The percutaneous technique described by Ma and Griffith was used, and it was found that the sural nerve had become proximally entrapped by the suture in three of five cases.[14,15] There was no sural nerve entrapment in the open cases.[14]

Incidence with Different Techniques

Percutaneous

Ma and Griffith's percutaneous technique is one of the most widely reported.[15] In their original series, along with the subsequent studies of Ceccarelli and colleagues[16] and Bradley and Tibone,[14,15,17] there was no sural nerve involvement reported, despite Hockenbury's findings. Other authors have reported rates between 3% and 40% using this and other percutaneous techniques.[8,18–22] With entirely percutaneous techniques, the sural nerve is not visualized, and it inevitably is placed at risk during passage of the suture. Small stab incisions with blunt dissection to the tendon and retraction may lower the risk slightly, but, given the variable course of the nerve, it is not possible to guarantee the suture will not entrap it. It is also possible that sural nerve complications may be under reported as, although they can have very troubling symptoms, many patients just have reduced sensation that may not be spontaneously reported. The symptoms from sural nerve entrapment also may be self-limiting. Using a modified Ma and Griffith repair, Haji and colleagues[20] had a 10.5% sural nerve involvement rate that resolved spontaneously during the follow up period.

Miniopen/minimally invasive

To reduce the potential for nerve entrapment, other authors have developed miniopen techniques that either attempt to identify the sural nerve laterally or avoid it altogether by staying in the midline.[10,23] Lansdaal and colleagues[23] reported on a minimally invasive surgical technique in which they visualized and spared the sural nerve. In spite of this, 9.2% of patients had sensory loss in its distribution, although most did not consider it uncomfortable. Webb used three transverse incisions, the distal two in the midline, and the proximal incision just over the medial half of the TA to reduce the chance of sural nerve injury. They had no sural nerve involvement in 27 patients.[10]

Open

Open techniques are not free from sural nerve complication either. Reported rates vary between 0% and 20%.[9,17,20,21,24–30] In Nistor's study, 9 of 45 patients (20%) following an open repair had sural nerve symptoms; in seven of these cases, a lateral incision had been used.[30] A medial incision therefore is recommended when undertaking an open repair.

Conservative

The authors have been unable to identify any sural nerve complications following conservative treatment. In theory, iatrogenic injury to the sural nerve is avoided, although the potential for compressive neuropathy from poorly fitting casts exists. An interesting observation from the study by Lim and colleagues[8] was that 7 of 66 patients reported paresthesia in the sural nerve distribution before treatment for a TA rupture, indicating a concomitant injury to the nerve. It therefore is recommended that patients be assessed specifically for sural nerve dysfunction before treatment, particularly if operative repair is being considered.

WOUND HEALING PROBLEMS
Introduction

Wound healing problems can be common following operative treatment of Achilles tendon disorders. They range from minor complications, such as adhesions, to major complications with deep infection associated with wound breakdown and tendon necrosis. The rate is influenced by the technique chosen, but it is difficult to make direct comparisons because of the lack of definition of the types of complication when reported.

Influence of Technique

In a quantitative review, Wong and colleagues[31] divided complications into minor and major groups following conservative, percutaneous, and open repairs, also differentiating between early mobilization and immobilization. They found open repair with immobilization to have the highest rate of minor wound complications (12.3%) compared with percutaneous (4.9%) and conservative repairs (0.5%). Early mobilization reduced the rate in the open group to 4.9% but increased it slightly in the percutaneous group (6.6%). The complications in the conservative group were all adhesions from direct trauma at the time of injury. Khan and colleagues,[7] in their meta-analysis, showed a significant reduction in the complication rate comparing functional bracing with immobilization ($P = .001$), particularly with respect to adhesion formation. This effect also was demonstrated by Mortensen and colleagues,[29] who showed that early mobilization following an open TA repair resulted in fewer and less severe adhesions ($P = .01$).

Although there are concerns regarding sural nerve injury using percutaneous techniques in TA repair, there is a clear benefit in terms of wound healing. Several authors have reported no wound complications following percutaneous repair.[8,15–17,21,32] Lim and colleagues[8] found a wound infection rate of 21% and an adhesion rate of 6% following open TA repair and 0% for each, using a percutaneous technique. Haji and colleagues[20] found a deep infection rate of 5.7% and 0% when comparing open and percutaneous repair.

Risk Factors

Bruggeman and colleagues[33] specifically examined wound complications following open repair of TA ruptures and made an analysis of the risk factors. Of the 164 patients retrospectively reviewed, 10.4% developed a wound complication. Tobacco use ($P<.0001$, risk ratio [RR] 8.1), steroids ($P<.0005$, RR 6.8), and female sex ($P = .04$, RR 2.7) were identified as statistically significant, independent, risk factors for wound healing problems. Although diabetes was not an independent risk factor, a further increase in the complication rate was seen when combined with tobacco or steroids. Age, time to surgery, and body mass index (BMI) were not risk factors for wound complication.

Sorrenti, however, demonstrated a significant difference in the complication rate when comparing repair of acute, subacute, and chronic ruptures using a V-Y technique. The infection rates were 13%, 33%, and 43%, respectively.[34]

Angiosomes

Angiosomes play an important role when considering surgical approaches in the foot and ankle, and an in-depth review is provided by Attinger and colleagues.[35] An incision placed in the midline over the TA in theory, should be well placed for wound healing. The lateral side of such an incision is supplied by the peroneal angiosome and the medial side by the posterior tibial angiosome.[35] Also, provided the tibial and peroneal arteries are patent, there should be no problem with healing of an incision to either side of the midline.[35] Miniopen techniques often combine a short, transverse incision over the TA rupture with a percutaneous suture technique. Again, these incisions are well placed when considering the pattern of the angiosomes.[35]

Splinting the ankle in marked equinus may affect wound healing. Poynton and O'Rourke measured transcutaneous skin oxygen pressure (tcPO$_2$) in normal healthy volunteers and found it was best at 20° plantarflexion and worst with plantarflexion to 40°.[36] This may partially explain the lower wound complication rate in repairs that undergo early mobilization.[7,31]

Treatment

Major wound breakdown, skin loss, and tendon necrosis can pose a significant problem. To reconstruct the tendon, several techniques are available that are covered in reviews by Feibel, Maffulli, and Myerson,[11,37,38] and in this issue by Lin. Soft tissue cover is more problematic, as there is often not a suitable bed for a split-thickness skin graft, necessitating the use of techniques further up the reconstructive ladder. These include local pedicle flaps and free flaps, usually the radial forearm or latissimus dorsi muscle free flap (**Fig. 6**). Reconstruction of such defects should be performed in conjunction with a plastic surgeon.

CHANGES IN TENDON MORPHOLOGY

Tendon thickening following treatment of a TA rupture is common. Several authors have made particular comment on this finding, and although it is difficult to compare results directly, with measurements taken at different levels using different techniques, one can conclude that virtually all patients will have thickening of the injured TA regardless of the mode of treatment. Leppilahti and colleagues,[39] using ultrasound (US) assessment, found mean increases of 44%, 131%, and 237% in terms of tendon width, thickness, and cross-sectional area, respectively following an open repair. Maffulli and colleagues[40] and Kraus and colleagues[41] had similar findings, assessed again using US. The technique of repair may influence the degree of thickening; Bradley and Tibone compared percutaneous and open repairs, and while both groups showed tendon thickening, this was less marked in the percutaneous group (0.42 cm) than the open group (0.72 cm).[17] Nistor, however, showed no difference in tendon thickening when comparing open repair and conservative management, with a mean increase of 7 mm in both groups.[30] None of these studies have shown any correlation between thickening and clinical outcome.

Tendon calcification, however, can be symptomatic. Using US assessment, calcification was identified in 13% to 62% of patients following TA rupture.[39–41] Kraus and colleagues[41] found calcifications in 28% (10 of 26 patients), four of which were peritendinous and six intratendinous, ranging in size from 3 to 37 mm. Lesions over

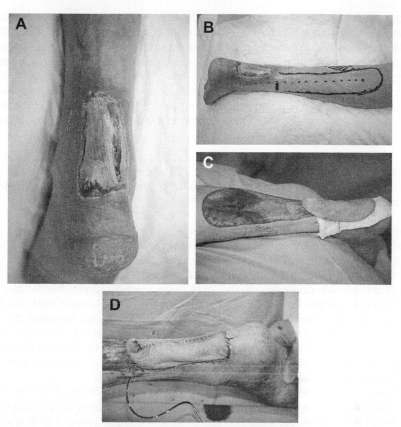

Fig. 6. Clinical photographs of local flap cover for skin loss and tendon necrosis, which was the result of deep wound infection following a decompression for tendonopathy. (*A*) Following a previous debridement, there is skin loss and necrotic tendon exposed. (*B*) Sural island flap marked out. (*C*) Flap mobilized and turned down, following tendon debridement and reconstruction with strip of fascia-lata. (*D*) Flap sutured and split skin graft applied to donor site.

10 mm in size tended to be symptomatic and associated with chronic swelling, decreased range of motion, and increased pain. They were unable to identify any risk factors for its development.

THROMBOEMBOLIC
Background

It is beyond the scope of this article to explore the controversies of venous thromboembolism (VTE) and its prophylaxis. The debate on thromboprophylaxis continues to gain momentum, with increased public awareness and the issue of often contradictory guidelines from different regulatory bodies: in the United States the American Association of Chest Physicians (AACP) and in the United Kingdom the National Institute for Clinical Excellence (NICE), along with guidelines produced by the Cochrane Collaboration.

Guidelines

The ACCP recommendation is "for patients with isolated lower-extremity injuries distal to the knee, we suggest that clinicians do not routinely use thromboprophylaxis."[42] This is at odds with the recommendations of the Cochrane Review; in a meta-analysis of six randomized controlled trials, they showed a significant reduction in the rate of Deep Vein Thrombosis (DVT) in patients immobilized in a cast for soft tissue injuries, detected by venography, phlebography, or US. They recommend that "low molecular weight heparin (LMWH) should be considered in patients...with a below knee cast."[43] In the United Kingdom, generic guidelines from NICE recommend mechanical prophylaxis and LMWH in patients undergoing orthopedic surgery.[44] More detailed, context-specific guidelines are being developed in conjunction with the British Orthopedic Association.

Rates

It is difficult to accurately establish the rate of VTE following TA rupture treatment. Only symptomatic DVTs tend to be reported, and it is difficult to compare studies with different immobilization regimes, no record of patient risk factors, or thromboprophylaxis.

In a double-blind, placebo-controlled trial of an LMWH, Lassen and colleagues[45] demonstrated a DVT rate of 9% in patients receiving the LMWH and 19% in the control group. The study group had been immobilized in a cast or brace following a TA rupture or leg fracture. They noted that TA ruptures were significantly more common in the LMWH group and did not differentiate between surgical and conservative treatment. There were 2 of 221 proven pulmonary embolisms, both in the placebo group. Similar rates are evident in the Cochrane Review, with an 11.8% and 19.1% DVT rate in the LMWH and control groups, respectively (cases treated with a below knee cast, operated or not).[43]

Lo and colleagues, in a quantitative review of TA ruptures, found a DVT rate of 1 of 701 ruptures (0.1%) in the operatively treated group and 4 of 248 (1.6%) in the nonoperative group. The PE rate was lower, with 0 of 701 (0%) in the operative group and 1 of 248 (0.4%) in the nonoperative group.[12]

The discrepancy between studies that only report the symptomatic DVTs and those that actively investigate for both symptomatic and asymptomatic DVT suggest that most DVTs following TA rupture are clinically silent. The significance of clinically silent DVTs remains subject to debate.

Summary

In the United States, the National Quality Forum recommend that every patient be assessed for his or her risk of VTE and that clinically appropriate, evidence-based methods of thromboprophylaxis be used.[46] In the absence of clinical guidelines based upon high quality evidence, however, the onus falls on the clinician to make a VTE risk assessment of each patient and treat each accordingly.

TENDON LENGTHENING POST TREATMENT OF ACHILLES RUPTURE
Introduction

The ability of muscles, through tendons, to carry out their function depends upon the tension within the musculotendinous unit. The muscles will have to contract to a greater degree to produce the same action if the musculotendinous unit is overly lengthened. This will lead to decreased power and, because of the additional effort required in attempting to produce this contractile force, decreased endurance. For advocates of surgical treatment, this simple physiologic basis has led to recommendations that

> "it is impossible to anatomically restore the correct length of the Achilles tendon with non-operative care.....if it is used, it should be done judiciously and rarely in the competitive athlete."[47]

There are varied results in the published literature, however, and lengthening after TA rupture is certainly a complication recognized in both operative and nonoperative studies.

Incidence

Lea and Smith were strong advocates of nonoperative management of Achilles tendon rupture because of high, previously published, rates of postoperative complications.[48] Range of movement measurements were available in 41 of their 55 patients. Eight patients had a 0° to 5° increase in dorsiflexion; eight had a 6° to 10° increase, and one patient had a 20° increase in dorsiflexion.

McComis and colleagues[49] reported on a series of 15 patients who were treated conservatively with functional bracing and had a mean follow-up of 31 months. They found that there was a statistically significant relationship between increased passive dorsiflexion of the ankle and vertical force output during gait. The actual measured difference was 2.6°. This, however, was not associated with any loss of performance.

Mortensen and colleagues[29] performed a prospective study of regimes of immobilization following surgical repair (conventional plaster treatment versus early functional bracing). They placed small steel sutures into the tendon ends so that separation could be measured radiographically. They found almost identical separation in both groups with a median of 11.5 mm (range 0 to 33 mm). They had almost identical strength index results in both groups (as compared with the uninjured side) of between 0.75 and 0.89 dependant upon foot position. There was no correlation between the degree of separation and the results of the strength tests. These results show significant separation, and this may have been partially contributed to by the aggressiveness of their postoperative regimes. Cetti and colleagues[50] also studied the effect of a mobile cast versus a rigid cast in surgically treated patients. They found (using surgically placed radiographic monitors) a mean elongation of 6.1 mm in the mobile cast group and of 13.5 mm in the rigid cast group.

Nistor performed a prospective randomized study into surgical and nonsurgical treatment of primary Achilles tendon ruptures.[30] He reported that changes in range of motion after both types of treatment were small. Sixty-six percent of surgical patients and 74% of nonsurgical patients had changes of less than 5°. Thirty-four percent of surgical patients had changes of 10° or more, although these tended to be restrictions in plantarflexion. Twenty six percent of nonsurgical patients had changes of 10° or more, and these tended to be a small restriction in plantarflexion with an increase in dorsiflexion. All patients, however, were able to walk on tiptoe, although many of these had differences in the heel height that was achievable. On formal testing with a dynamometer, there were no differences between the groups.

Moller and colleagues[51] also reported a prospective randomized study comparing surgical and nonsurgical management. They reported an increase in dorsiflexion in 42% of surgically treated patients and in 48% on the nonsurgically treated patients. There were no significant differences in isometric testing between the two groups. Two years after injury, 69% of the endurance had been recovered in the surgical group compared with 54% in the nonsurgical group. Eight percent of the surgical group and 22% of the nonsurgical group were unable to perform a single heel raise 2 years after injury.

From the limited data available, it seems clear that elongation occurs with all treatment and mobilization protocols. The data suggest, however, that this is less in surgically treated patients who undergo early functional mobilization programs. This should be an area for further robust investigation.

Treatment

In the authors' experience, elongation of the Achilles tendon following treatment of a rupture only tends to be symptomatic in the higher functioning athlete, unless there has been a complication of treatment with ensuing excessive elongation. There is a paucity of published literature on the treatment of this condition. One small series reported by Cannon and Hackney[52] showed good success. All five patients presented with an impairment of previous sporting activity, and all returned to their chosen level of sporting activity after surgical treatment. The surgical method used was a Z shortening. The authors have used this technique successfully but only have resorted to this technique if the quality of the tendon is suspect on MRI. If the tendon morphology appears relatively normal, then an end-to-end repair is performed via a miniopen percutaneous technique. The authors have not found it necessary to augment the repair with a tendon transfer, as the tendon should be functionally normal if the correct length is restored. This also avoids the extra bulk of the transfer and possible symptoms from the harvested site. The most critical step in avoiding this condition is restoring the correct length at the index operation. It is often, therefore, advisable to prepare and drape both legs with the feet hanging off the table during the procedure. Correct tension then may be assured by comparing the degree of plantar flexion of both feet.

COMPLEX REGIONAL PAIN SYNDROME

Complex regional pain syndrome (CRPS) is a condition characterized by abnormal pain, swelling, and vasomotor instability and later stiffness and joint contracture. CRPS type 1 develops after a noxious event, for example a TA rupture, and type 2 develops after a nerve injury (eg, sural nerve entrapment). It previously has been known by several different names, most commonly reflex sympathetic dystrophy or Sudek atrophy. Despite its predilection for the hand and foot, it rarely is described following a TA rupture. The authors have identified only two articles that report single cases following treatment of a TA rupture. Webb and Bannister reported one case (1 of 27) following treatment with using a percutaneous repair and Nada a single case (1 of 33) following external fixation of a TA rupture.[10,53] Although the incidence of mild cases is probably under-reported, going unrecognized, or resolving with physiotherapy, the rate of severe chronic CRPS is very low.

COMPARTMENT SYNDROME

The authors have not identified any reported cases of compartment syndrome directly attributed to a TA rupture. Reed and Hiemstra reported a single patient who developed anterior compartment syndrome following a standard open Achilles tendon repair. The cause of this was unclear, but factors considered were: patient positioning, pneumatic tourniquet, vasospasm, and anatomic abnormality.[54]

SUMMARY

Treatment of the Achilles tendon has been fraught with complications since the time of Hippocrates. After initial enthusiasm for operative treatment in the late 18th and early 19th centuries, the complication rates of surgery led to doyennes of orthopedic surgery steering toward nonoperative management. The advent of modern techniques and better understanding of pathogenesis of the Achilles tendon have led to resurgence in the popularity of operative treatment. The spectrum of complications differs between operative and nonoperative treatments. Rerupture, elongation of the tendon (and diminished function), and tendon thickening may occur with either technique, although rates seem to be higher with nonoperative management. The incidence and significance of venous thromboembolism are uncertain, and coherent guidelines are not available. Wound problems (providing sufficient care is taken with nonoperative management) and sural nerve morbidity should occur only with operative treatment. The authors believe that the overall incidence of all these complications from surgery is lessened with percutaneous/miniopen techniques. Whether nonoperative or operative treatment is utilized, there is robust evidence that early functional, but controlled, mobilization provides better results.

Absolute polarization toward either operative or nonoperative treatment is not clinically sound. Appropriate informed consent needs to be undertaken. This must take into account the patient's level of activity and wishes coupled with an understanding of their comorbidities and the effects that they will have upon complication rates.

REFERENCES

1. Homer. The Iliad. Nagles R, translator-editor. New York: Viking; 1996.
2. Carden D, Noble J, Chalmers J, et al. Rupture of the calcaneal tendon. The early and late management. J Bone Joint Surg Br 1987;69(3):416–20.
3. Carlstedt CA. Mechanical and chemical factors in tendon healing. Effects of indomethacin and surgery in the rabbit. Acta Orthop Scand Suppl 1987;224:1–75.
4. Klenerman L. The early history of tendo Achillis and its rupture. J Bone Joint Surg Br 2007;89(4):545–7.
5. Pajala A, Kangas J, Ohtonen P, et al. Rerupture and deep infection following treatment of total Achilles tendon rupture. J Bone Joint Surg Am 2002,84(11).2016–21.
6. Bhandari M, Guyatt GH, Siddiqui F, et al. Treatment of acute Achilles tendon ruptures: a systematic overview and meta-analysis. Clin Orthop Relat Res 2002;400:190–200.
7. Khan RJK, Fick D, Keogh A, et al. Treatment of acute Achilles tendon ruptures. A meta-analysis of randomized, controlled trials. J Bone Joint Surg Am 2005;87(10): 2202–10.
8. Lim J, Dalal R, Waseem M. Percutaneous vs. open repair of the ruptured Achilles tendon—a prospective randomized controlled study. Foot Ankle Int 2001;22(7): 559–68.
9. Wagnon R, Akayi M. The Webb-Bannister percutaneous technique for acute Achilles' tendon ruptures: a functional and MRI assessment. J Foot Ankle Surg 2005;44(6):437–44.
10. Webb JM, Bannister GC. Percutaneous repair of the ruptured tendo Achillis. J Bone Joint Surg Br 1999;81(5):877–80.
11. Maffulli N, Ajis A. Management of chronic ruptures of the Achilles tendon. J Bone Joint Surg Am 2008;90(6):1348–60.
12. Lo IK, Kirkley A, Nonweiler B, et al. Operative versus nonoperative treatment of acute Achilles tendon ruptures: a quantitative review. Clin J Sport Med 1997; 7(3):207–11.
13. Webb J, Moorjani N, Radford M. Anatomy of the sural nerve and its relation to the Achilles tendon. Foot Ankle Int 2000;21(6):475–7.
14. Hockenbury RT, Johns JC. A biomechanical in vitro comparison of open versus percutaneous repair of tendon Achilles. Foot Ankle 1990;11(2):67–72.
15. Ma GW, Griffith TG. Percutaneous repair of acute closed ruptured Achilles tendon: a new technique. Clin Orthop Relat Res 1977;(128):247–55.

16. Ceccarelli F, Berti L, Giuriati L, et al. Percutaneous and minimally invasive techniques of Achilles tendon repair. Clin Orthop Relat Res 2007;458:188–93.
17. Bradley JP, Tibone JE. Percutaneous and open surgical repairs of Achilles tendon ruptures. A comparative study. Am J Sports Med 1990;18(2):188–95.
18. Buchgraber A, Pässler HH. Percutaneous repair of Achilles tendon rupture. Immobilization versus functional postoperative treatment. Clin Orthop Relat Res 1997;(341):113–22.
19. Cretnik A, Kosanović M, Smrkolj V. Percutaneous suturing of the ruptured Achilles tendon under local anesthesia. J Foot Ankle Surg 2004;43(2):72–81.
20. Haji A, Sahai A, Symes A, et al. Percutaneous versus open tendo Achillis repair. Foot Ankle Int 2004;25(4):215–8.
21. Goren D, Ayalon M, Nyska M. Isokinetic strength and endurance after percutaneous and open surgical repair of Achilles tendon ruptures. Foot Ankle Int 2005;26(4):286–90.
22. Rowley DI, Scotland TR. Rupture of the Achilles tendon treated by a simple operative procedure. Injury 1982;14(3):252–4.
23. Lansdaal JR, Goslings JC, Reichart M, et al. The results of 163 Achilles tendon ruptures treated by a minimally invasive surgical technique and functional after treatment. Injury 2007;38(7):839–44.
24. Andersen E, Hvass I. Suture of Achilles tendon rupture under local anesthesia. Acta Orthop Scand 1986;57(3):235–6.
25. Cetti R, Christensen SE, Ejsted R, et al. Operative versus nonoperative treatment of Achilles tendon rupture. A prospective randomized study and review of the literature. Am J Sports Med 1993;21(6):791–9.
26. Jaakkola JI, Beskin JL, Griffith LH, et al. Early ankle motion after triple bundle technique repair vs. casting for acute Achilles tendon rupture. Foot Ankle Int 2001;22(12):979–84.
27. Jessing P, Hansen E. Surgical treatment of 102 tendo Achillis ruptures—suture or tenontoplasty? Acta Chir Scand 1975;141(5):370–7.
28. Kellam JF, Hunter GA, McElwain JP. Review of the operative treatment of Achilles tendon rupture. Clin Orthop Relat Res 1985;(201):80–3.
29. Mortensen HM, Skov O, Jensen PE. Early motion of the ankle after operative treatment of a rupture of the Achilles tendon. A prospective, randomized clinical and radiographic study. J Bone Joint Surg Am 1999;81(7):983–90.
30. Nistor L. Surgical and nonsurgical treatment of Achilles tendon rupture. A prospective randomized study. J Bone Joint Surg Am 1981;63(3):394–9.
31. Wong J, Barrass V, Maffulli N. Quantitative review of operative and nonoperative management of Achilles tendon ruptures. Am J Sports Med 2002;30(4):565–75.
32. Atherton W, Dangas S, Henry A. Advantages of semiclosed over open method of repair of ruptured Achilles tendon. Foot Ankle Surg 2000;6:27–30.
33. Bruggeman N, Turner N, Dahm D, et al. Wound complications after open Achilles tendon repair: an analysis of risk factors. Clin Orthop Relat Res 2004;427:63–6.
34. Sorrenti SJ. Achilles tendon rupture: effect of early mobilization in rehabilitation after surgical repair. Foot Ankle Int 2006;27(6):407–10.
35. Attinger C, Cooper P, Blume P, et al. The safest surgical incisions and amputations applying the angiosome principles and using the Doppler to assess the arterial–arterial connections of the foot and ankle. Foot Ankle Clin 2001;6(4):745–99.
36. Poynton AR, O'Rourke K. An analysis of skin perfusion over the Achilles tendon in varying degrees of plantarflexion. Foot Ankle Int 2001;22(7):572–4.

37. Feibel JB, Bernacki BL. A review of salvage procedures after failed Achilles tendon repair. Foot Ankle Clin 2003;8(1):105–14.
38. Myerson MS. Achilles tendon ruptures. Instr Course Lect 1999;48:219–30.
39. Leppilahti J, Forsman K, Puranen J, et al. Outcome and prognostic factors of Achilles rupture repair using a new scoring method. Clin Orthop Relat Res 1998;346:152–61.
40. Maffulli N, Tallon C, Wong J, et al. Early weight bearing and ankle mobilization after open repair of acute midsubstance tears of the Achilles tendon. Am J Sports Med 2003;31(5):692–700.
41. Kraus R, Stahl J, Meyer C, et al. Frequency and effects of intratendinous and peritendinous calcifications after open Achilles tendon repair. Foot Ankle Int 2004;25(11):827–32.
42. Hirsh J, Guyatt G, Albers GW, et al. Executive summary: American College of Chest Physicians evidence-based clinical practice guidelines 8th edition. Chest 2008;133(Suppl 6):71S–109S.
43. Testroote M, Stigter W, de Visser DC, et al. Low molecular weight heparin for prevention of venous thromboembolism in patients with lower-leg immobilization. Cochrane Database Syst Rev 2008;(4):CD006681.
44. Royal College of Surgeons of England. Venous thromboembolism: reducing the risk in surgical patients. London: National Collaborating Centre for Acute Care; 2007.
45. Lassen MR, Borris LC, Nakov RL. Use of the low molecular weight heparin reviparin to prevent deep-vein thrombosis after leg injury requiring immobilization. N Engl J Med 2002;347(10):726–30.
46. Meyer GS, Denham CR, Angood PB, et al. Safe practices for better healthcare–2009 update: a consensus report. Washington, DC: National Quality Forum (NQF) 2009.
47. Soma CA, Mandelbaum BR. Repair of acute Achilles tendon ruptures. Orthop Clin North Am 1995;26(2):239–47.
48. Lea RB, Smith L. Nonsurgical treatment of tendo Achillis rupture. J Bone Joint Surg Am 1972;54(7):1398–407.
49. McComis GP, Nawoczenski DA, DeHaven KE. Functional bracing for rupture of the Achilles tendon. Clinical results and analysis of ground reaction forces and temporal data. J Bone Joint Surg Am 1997;79(12):1799–808.
50. Cetti R, Henriksen LO, Jacobsen KS. A new treatment of ruptured Achilles tendons. A prospective randomized study. Clin Orthop Relat Res 1994;308:155–65.
51. Möller M, Movin T, Granhed H, et al. Acute rupture of tendon Achillis. A prospective randomised study of comparison between surgical and nonsurgical treatment. J Bone Joint Surg Br 2001;83(6):843–8.
52. Cannon LB, Hackney RG. Operative shortening of the elongated defunctioned tendoachillies following previous rupture. J R Nav Med Serv 2003;89(3):139–41.
53. Nada A. Rupture of the calcaneal tendon. Treatment by external fixation. J Bone Joint Surg Br 1985;67(3):449–53.
54. Reed J, Hiemstra LA. Anterior compartment syndrome following an Achilles tendon repair: an unusual complication. Clin J Sport Med 2004;14(4):237–41.

Posterior Calf Injury

John T. Campbell, MD

KEYWORDS

• Calf injury • Calf strain • Gastrocnemius • Soleus • Plantaris

Acute injuries of the Achilles tendon are common among athletes and nonathletes alike. Injuries of the other posterior calf muscles are far less common but should be considered in the differential, to ensure proper diagnosis and treatment of patients with calf injuries. This article focuses on these calf injuries, including injuries of the gastrocnemius, plantaris, soleus, and flexor hallucis longus (FHL) muscles, which may occasionally be mistaken for Achilles tendon disorders.

GASTROCNEMIUS INJURY ("TENNIS LEG")

Gastrocnemius muscle strain or rupture causes posterior calf pain that can mimic Achilles tendon pathology. The gastrocnemius is particularly susceptible to injury because of its position spanning across 3 joints: the knee, ankle, and subtalar.[1–3] The medial head arises from the medial femoral condyle, whereas the lateral head originates from the posterior aspect of the lateral femoral condyle.[4] The mechanism of injury involves stretching of the muscle during eccentric contraction,[5] as occurs when the ankle is forced into dorsiflexion while the knee is extended.[1–3,6–17] Gastrocnemius strain occurs most commonly in middle-aged or older patients,[1,2,7,10–13,18–20] and may be related to physiologic changes of muscle with aging.[2,16,19] Loss of flexibility may predispose to muscle injury.[2,5,16,17] Gastrocnemius strain may also occur in younger athletes, as evidenced by the common eponym of "tennis leg" that is used to describe rupture of the medial head of the gastrocnemius at the musculotendinous junction.[1–3,12,14,15,17] Less common is rupture of the lateral head of the gastrocnemius.[12,20] Gastrocnemius strain may occur during warm-up activity or later due to muscle fatigue with impaired coordination.[5,20] Gastrocnemius injury commonly happens during racquet sports, running, basketball, football, and skiing.[8,10,11,13] One report also described this injury happening during namaz prayer, when the individual kneels and lies with the head prostrate on the ground; the muscle is then eccentrically stretched when the individual arises with the hands positioned on the knees as they extend.[16]

The patient typically complains of acute onset of pain in the proximal calf.[3,6,9,10,12–14,17,18,21] The anatomic proximity may suggest proximal Achilles tendon strain, as can the oft-described sensation of tearing, popping, or feeling as if the calf has been kicked or struck by a ball or racquet.[1–3,7,10,13–16,20] Some patients recall

---

Institute for Foot and Ankle Reconstruction at Mercy, 301 St Paul Place, Baltimore, MD 21202, USA
E-mail address: jcampbell@mdmercy.com

Foot Ankle Clin N Am 14 (2009) 761–771
doi:10.1016/j.fcl.2009.07.005
1083-7515/09/$ – see front matter © 2009 Elsevier Inc. All rights reserved.

prodromal symptoms of calf pain before the injury[2,3,7,13,14,17]; one series reported this in 20% of patients.[13] Pain, cramping, muscle weakness, ecchymosis, and significant swelling are the norm[2,3,7–9,17]; such findings may be mistaken for a deep vein thrombosis.[1,3,7,9–11,15–17] Patients often have difficulty ambulating.[1,2,12] Several authors have cautioned about empiric use of anticoagulants before confirmation of a thrombosis, as this may lead to hemorrhage and hematoma in the leg.[1,7,10,11,14,17] In rare cases, severe bleeding and hematoma formation can precipitate a compartment syndrome of the calf.[1,3,7,10,11,14,17]

On physical examination, the patient is tender over the muscle tear.[9,15,20] On palpation, the area of muscle strain may remain in continuity[21] or a rupture may be palpable if there is frank retraction of the site.[1,3,7,10,12,14,15,20] It may be difficult to distinguish this muscle tear clinically from a tear of the Achilles tendon, particularly if the proximal aspect of that tendon is involved.[20] The patient may have pain with passive stretch of the calf or with resistance to plantar flexion.[1,19,20] It is important to rule out clinical findings of compartment syndrome, such as an extremely tense muscle compartment, severe pain with passive motion of the ankle, or impaired neurovascular function.

Radiologic studies can assist in diagnosis, particularly in differentiating between partial and complete ruptures. Plain radiographs and computed tomography scans are of limited use in this soft tissue injury. As with other muscle strains, ultrasound is an effective tool for diagnosing gastrocnemius injury.[6,16] This offers the advantage of nonionizing radiation and is relatively inexpensive.[6] Ultrasound findings include disruption of the normal fiber alignment at the musculotendinous junction,[6,10,11,16] hematoma,[6,10] and fluid collection between the gastrocnemius and soleus muscles.[10,11,16,18] This technique can also differentiate partial tears from complete tears of the muscle, with reports indicating that the incidence of partial injuries ranges between one-third and three-quarters of cases.[6,10,11,16] Ultrasound can determine the size of the associated hematoma, with a larger dimension correlated with complete rupture rather than partial tear.[10] Ultrasound can also determine the size of the defect in a complete rupture and has been used to guide percutaneous aspiration of the hematoma, although this typically recurs.[6] Ultrasound can also be performed to rule out the presence of a deep vein thrombosis, clarifying an otherwise confusing clinical picture.[10,15,18] With its low cost and ease of use, ultrasound can also assess later healing; features include progressive decrease in the size of a hematoma, reparative tissue signified by a peripheral hypoechoic area that extends toward the center, and healing of muscle fibers by about 4 weeks.[10,11]

Magnetic resonance imaging (MRI) has become ubiquitous and offers superb soft tissue imaging. Findings include rupture or discontinuity of muscle fibers,[3,21] fluid signal consistent with hemorrhage and hematoma at the musculotendinous junction,[3,19,21] and retraction of the torn muscle fibers (**Fig. 1**).[3] MRI also allows differentiation between gastrocnemius and Achilles tendon injury, which can help to improve direct treatment.

Gastrocnemius injuries have a relatively benign prognosis.[2,7,13,15,17] Strains or partial tears often recover faster than complete ruptures. Early treatment focuses on symptomatic relief, including rest, ice treatment, compression wrapping, and elevation to minimize swelling (RICE).[1,8–11,13,15,17,19,20] Pharmacologic agents may be needed to provide analgesia and reduce muscle spasm, which can facilitate early commencement of stretching exercises.[7,8,10,11,13,14,20] The patient is allowed to ambulate as tolerated and to gradually increase activity level as symptoms subside.[7,14,15] Severe strains, however, may limit weight bearing and require resting of the limb with a cast or boot orthosis. The patient can advance weight bearing and dorsiflexion stretching once symptoms subside.[8,15]

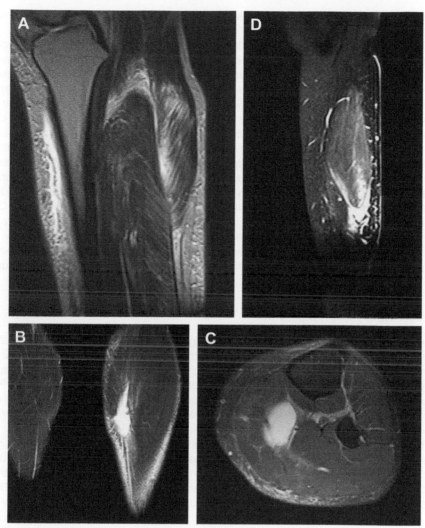

Fig. 1. (*A*) MRI sagittal T2 image showing edema and discontinuity of gastrocnemius muscle fibers. (*B*) Coronal and (*C*) axial T2 images showing hematoma at gastrocnemius musculo-tendinous junction. (*D*) Sagittal image indicating retraction of muscle fibers consistent with complete gastrocnemius rupture. (*Courtesy of* John Carrino, MD, MPH.)

Physical therapy has an important role in facilitating recovery. Early interventions include gentle calf stretching, massage, and cryotherapy.[10,11,13,17,19] Subsequently, strength training, heel raises, proprioception training, and closed-chain exercises are added along with core strengthening and general conditioning.[10,11,13] Patients will resume running, jumping, and cutting sports once they are pain free and demonstrate normal strength and agility. This may take up to 3 to 4 months.[7,10,11,21]

Surgical treatment is rarely described.[12] Older reports discussed repair of the muscle tear.[12] However, such repair is technically challenging because of the difficulty with suture fixation through muscle tissue along with the potential for fibrosis and contracture at the site. Appropriate indications for surgical repair remain ill defined in contemporary literature due to the successful outcomes noted with nonoperative management.

Good-quality evidence-based literature on gastrocnemius injuries is surprisingly sparse for such a common injury. Numerous case reports (level V) discuss gastrocnemius tears ("tennis leg"), highlighting their benign nature and generally good prognosis for resolution of pain, functional recovery, and return to sports.[1,14,21] One level IV retrospective case series described 25 patients who sustained a gastrocnemius tear and were followed clinically for 1 to 3 years.[13] These patients were treated nonoperatively with a compression sleeve, heel lift, ice, and antiinflammatory medications. Subsequently, the patients advanced to calf stretches, isometric and resistance strengthening, and toe raises. The group had a mean convalescence time of 4.5 weeks and a mean time of 6.7 weeks to return to sports. All patients resumed preinjury sports pursuits. Cybex plantar flexion strength testing at a mean time of 27 months postinjury revealed no significant difference between the injured and the noninjured limbs. On sequential Cybex testing, 2 patients demonstrated normalization of strength by 6 months, prompting the authors to recommend continued strength training for 3 months, even after the patients had resumed sports.[13] As such, nonoperative treatment of these common injuries appears to offer good clinical outcomes and return to function.

PLANTARIS AND SOLEUS INJURIES

Injuries of the plantaris and soleus muscles are far less common than those of the gastrocnemius. Controversy did exist in the orthopedic literature regarding the existence of plantaris and soleus tears. Early descriptions of plantaris or soleus tears were later disputed, with several investigators questioning their existence.[2,12,22] Subsequently, the advent of modern imaging technology along with surgically documented lesions confirmed these entities.[23,24] Nonetheless, these are less commonly seen than the more frequent gastrocnemius injuries.[25]

The small plantaris muscle arises from the supracondylar ridge of the lateral femoral condyle and courses medially as it progresses down the leg to its insertion on the calcaneus, just medial to the Achilles tendon.[18,22,24,26] The plantaris muscle and tendon run between the overlying gastrocnemius and the deeper soleus.[18,22,24] The soleus muscle arises from the posterior aspect of the upper fibula, the soleal line of the posterior tibia, and the fibrous arch between the 2 bones.[4] Plantaris injuries occur after ankle dorsiflexion while the knee is extended, similar to gastrocnemius tears.[25] In contrast, soleus tears occur when the ankle is passively dorsiflexed while the knee is flexed,[25] because it does not cross both joints (as the gastrocnemius does). Injuries to the plantaris or soleus have been described during running[27] and volleyball,[25] whereas others have noted their occurrence with simply stepping off a curb or with no identifiable trauma.[23,26,28] Clinically, it may be difficult to distinguish among soleus, plantaris, and gastrocnemius injuries; further, all of these entities may mimic proximal Achilles tendon strain or tear. A series of 141 patients referred for ultrasound examination after calf strain revealed that 67% had gastrocnemius tears, 21% had hematoma and fluid accumulation but no clear muscle tear, 9% had deep vein thrombosis, 1.4% had plantaris rupture, and 0.7% had isolated soleus tear.[18] The patient with a plantaris or soleus injury has an acute onset of pain, swelling, and ecchymosis of the calf.[23,26,27] Pain is exacerbated with passive dorsiflexion of the ankle, and there is point tenderness over the area of injury.[25] Weight bearing may be painful,[26,27] although some authors suggest that pain and swelling are less because of the smaller size of these muscles compared with the gastrocnemius.[24,28] Deep vein thrombosis can occur with injury to these muscles, and compartment syndrome of the calf may be a concern.[24,26,27]

Diagnostic imaging of these injuries again relies on ultrasound and MRI scanning. Ultrasound offers a fast and inexpensive imaging modality to diagnose plantaris or soleus injuries. Such injuries may also be found on sonography obtained to rule out deep vein thrombosis, clarifying a potentially confusing clinical picture.[28,29] Comparison with the contralateral extremity can assist in detecting subtle differences.[28] Features seen on ultrasound include disruption or disorganization of the muscle fibers, along with fluid collection or hematoma between the gastrocnemius and soleus.[29] Fluid collection alone without obvious tear of the muscle fibers has also been described.[29] Plantaris tear is typically located at midcalf level at the muscle-tendon junction.[29] Less commonly, tear of the plantaris tendon without muscle involvement may show little fluid on ultrasound.[28] In cases of chronic tear, a solid mass consistent with fibrosis or granulation tissue is noted instead of acute hematoma.[29] MRI scanning is also helpful in diagnosing tears of the plantaris or soleus muscles.[23–25] It is helpful to compare the injured extremity with the contralateral leg to identify potential injury.[25] MRI features of plantaris injury include hemorrhage and edema in the muscle seen on T1 and T2 imaging[25]; this fluid is located between the gastrocnemius and soleus muscles (**Fig. 2**).[24] Soleus injuries occur throughout the extent of the muscle (**Fig. 3**), whereas plantaris injuries are usually localized to the musculotendinous junction.[24] Associated injuries described on MRI include rupture of the anterior cruciate ligament, the lateral head of the gastrocnemius, the soleus, and the popliteus muscles.[24]

Similar to strains or ruptures of the gastrocnemius muscle, nonoperative treatment is the mainstay. Rest, ice, compression, and elevation are initiated along with the use of antiinflammatory and analgesic medications for symptomatic relief.[25,26] Protected weight bearing with the use of crutches and a fracture boot orthosis or cast may be necessary if the patient is symptomatic enough.[25] As symptoms subside, the patient performs gentle stretching, strengthening, and balance exercises. Slow advancement of activity and resumption of sports should proceed once the patient is asymptomatic and has regained symmetric motion and strength. Surgical treatment is rarely

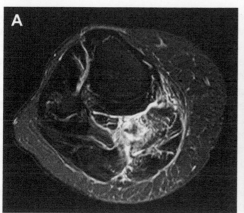
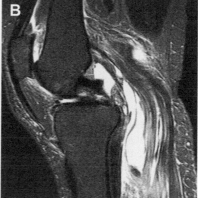

Fig. 2. (*A*) MRI axial fat suppression image of edema within plantaris muscle. (*B*) Sagittal T2 image of plantaris rupture, indicating fluid collection between gastrocnemius and soleus muscles with discontinuity at musculotendinous junction. (*Courtesy of* John Carrino, MD, MPH.)

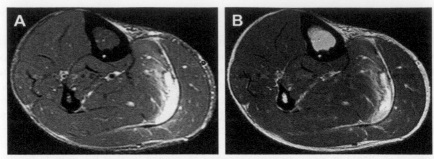

Fig. 3. (A) MRI T2 and (B) T1 axial images showing edema and hematoma within soleus muscle belly after strain. (*Courtesy of* John Carrino, MD, MPH.)

indicated for these injuries. One report on a surgically treated plantaris tear mentioned that the operation was performed due to concern for a possible neoplasm that was misidentified on the MRI scan[23]; another report confirmed tears of the plantaris and soleus muscles on surgical fasciotomies to relieve compartment syndrome of the calf.[27]

Based on the limited reports available, outcomes of plantaris and soleus tears are generally good. Case reports (level V) of plantaris ruptures indicated resolution of symptoms after a few weeks with either nonoperative management or surgical exploration.[23,28] However, these reports discuss only a few patients. One level V case report described a soleus tear in a volleyball player. Symptoms resolved after 4 weeks of cast immobilization, and the patient fully recovered without further complaints.[25] There is a paucity of good quality outcomes data on these uncommon injuries, so firm evidence-based recommendations are not yet available. Consequently, the author agrees with recommendations to pursue nonsurgical treatment for plantaris or soleus injuries.

FHL PATHOLOGY

Chronic FHL pathology is caused by stenosis of the tendon in its fibrous sheath posterior to the ankle, often in combination with posterior ankle impingement from an os trigonum.[30–38] Tenosynovitis, tendon thickening, nodularity, and even partial longitudinal tearing can occur in chronic cases.[31,34,36,39,40] Acute FHL injury is much less common,[41] resulting in tendon tear or strain at the musculotendinous junction or within the sheath adjacent to the talus.[42] Such acute injuries in the deep posterior calf or ankle may be confused with Achilles tendon tears and should be considered in the absence of classic findings of Achilles disruption. Other FHL injuries include those at the midfoot (at the knot of Henry), those at the plantar aspect of the hallux metatarsophalangeal joint, and the avulsion of the plantar aspect of the distal phalanx of the hallux[34,43,44]; these injuries are beyond the scope of this article, which focuses on posterior calf and ankle pathology.

The FHL muscle arises from the lower third of the posterior fibula and interosseous membrane.[34,35,45] The musculotendinous junction is at the level of the posterior ankle where the tendon enters a fibro-osseous tunnel between the medial and lateral posterior processes of the talus.[34,35] The tendon then passes inferiorly to the sustentaculum tali and crosses the flexor digitorum longus tendon at the knot of Henry in the midfoot.[34,35]

Unlike injuries of the other calf muscles, which occur with ankle dorsiflexion, acute injuries of the FHL have variable mechanisms. Hyperextension against resistance has been described,[42] as has been tearing, while pushing off with the forefoot planted during heel raise.[41] FHL injury along with concomitant Achilles tear has also been described.[42] Less-distinct mechanisms include painful giving way, snapping, or a "popping" sensation while walking or running, particularly if the athlete is training on hills.[35,44,45] Posterior impingement can occur while the ankle is plantarflexed (eg, kicking a ball or dancing *en pointe*).[31,32,36,39] Similar to other instances of degenerative tendinosis, an acute tear superimposed on a chronically damaged tendon can occur.[32]

Acute injuries of the FHL have been described in long-distance runners, divers, ballet dancers, soccer players, swimmers, and tennis and racquetball players.[32,35,41,43–45] Chronic FHL pathology occurs classically in dancers, but similar conditions do occur in runners and other nondancers.[30,34,36–40] Pain is localized to the posteromedial ankle, and a snapping sensation may be elicited while the ankle is dorsiflexed and the hallux interphalangeal joint is flexed.[31,34–36,39,45] Tenderness posterior to the medial malleolus is encountered,[31,32,34,36–38,40,41,46] although frank swelling or ecchymosis is rare because of the deep location of the FHL. Flexion strength of the hallux interphalangeal joint against manual resistance is assessed for weakness and compared with the uninjured foot.[32,40,42,45,46] In some cases, triggering or crepitus can occur due to thickening of the tendon[31,33,36,38,39]; such patients may have difficulty flexing the toe while the ankle is dorsiflexed. Due to impaired flexion of the hallux, the toe may extend and impinge within shoe wear during sports or running, leading to a subungual hematoma.[43,46] FHL pathology can be differentiated from pure posterior ankle impingement, which demonstrates posterolateral pain on passive plantarflexion of the ankle[30,33,37]; however, the 2 conditions can coexist.[30,32,35] Achilles tendon pathology is readily apparent with palpation of its subcutaneous location.[37]

Radiographs of the foot can rule out an FHL avulsion injury of the toe, but radiographs of the ankle rarely demonstrate any findings related to the musculotendinous injury.[42] Older literature describes computerized tomography as a means to assess soft tissue injuries, indicating subluxation or dislocation of the tendon behind the talus.[35] MRI offers superior soft tissue imaging and has become the mainstay of diagnosis of posterior calf injuries as discussed earlier. MRI can demonstrate loss of continuity of the muscle fibers or tendon along with fluid or pseudocyst within the FHL sheath on T2-weighted images (**Fig. 4**).[36,37] MRI can also show muscle hypertrophy and chronic intratendinous changes consistent with degeneration.[36,40]

As with other posterior calf muscle injuries, the treatment of acute FHL muscle injury is typically nonoperative because of the difficulty with suturing torn muscle. Partial FHL tendon tears are initially treated nonoperatively if active flexion of the toe is maintained.[45] This focuses on rest, antiinflammatory medications, and temporary immobilization. Physical therapy can be made beneficial by incorporating stretching, massage, and ultrasound techniques.[45] Complete FHL tears or partial injuries with severe weakness of toe flexion are addressed surgically to restore flexion power.[32,40–42,46] Surgery is also considered in cases of chronic FHL tenosynovitis that fails to respond to nonoperative means (**Fig. 5**).[30,31,33,34,36–39] A curvilinear incision is made posterior to the medial malleolus, and the flexor retinaculum is carefully divided.[31–33,36–39,41,42] The neurovascular bundle is identified in the tarsal tunnel and protected.[33,36,38,39,41] The FHL tendon sheath is then opened at the posterior ankle and extended distally to the level of the sustentaculum tali.[31,33,36,38,41,46] The tendon is inspected from the musculotendinous junction to the midfoot, and an associated os

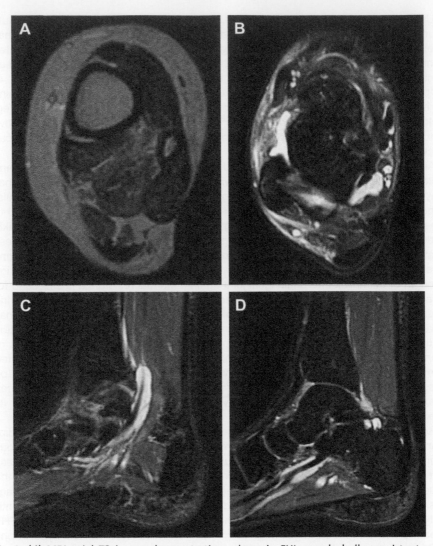

Fig. 4. (*A*) MRI axial T2 image demonstrating edema in FHL muscle belly consistent with muscle strain. (*B*) Axial fat suppression MRI image indicating pseudocyst of FHL sheath posterior to talus. Fat suppression sagittal images showing fluid within FHL sheath behind talus (*C*) and more distally along FHL tendon past sustentaculum tali (*D*). (*Courtesy of John Carrino, MD, MPH.*)

trigonum is excised to relieve potential impingement,[31,32,36] with the posterior talus smoothed using a rongeur and a rasp. Tenosynovectomy and debulking of the distal muscle fibers of the FHL may be necessary to eliminate stenosis and impingement within the sheath.[36,37,41] Partial tendon tears are debrided[34] and can be repaired with a running nonabsorbable suture.[31,36,41] Complete tears can be more challenging. Acute tears can be directly reapproximated and repaired with nonabsorbable core sutures under proper tension. Chronic complete tears may require debridement of

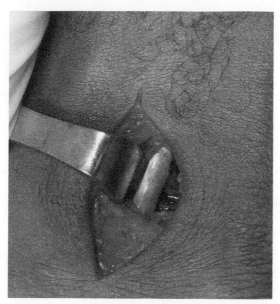

Fig. 5. Tenosynovitis of the FHL tendon. (*Courtesy of* Mark Myerson, MD.)

extensive tendon degeneration, precluding direct end-to-end repair; in such cases, side-to-side tenodesis to the flexor digitorum longus tendon has been described.[40,46] To bridge a large defect, reconstruction of the FHL has also been performed with tendon graft from the tensor fascia lata.[32] This author has no experience with that technique but would use a tendon allograft (such as a semitendinosus) if needed to restore FHL excursion and strength for hallux flexion. This is secured with nonabsorbable suture while the ankle is held in neutral dorsiflexion and the hallux is slightly flexed to tension properly.

Postoperatively, the muscle is kept non–weight bearing in a splint with a toe plate. Early literature describes immobilization in a short leg cast for up to 8 weeks.[32] Contemporary practice favors an early initiation of motion to prevent adhesions and to facilitate rehabilitation,[41,46] similar to repairs of the Achilles tendon. In cases involving pure tenolysis, debulking of the FHL muscle, os trigonum excision, or repair of a partial tendon tear, the patient can start active range of motion exercises and partial weight bearing in a boot orthosis after 2 weeks. After repair of complete tears, use of a boot orthosis with an extension block is helpful to avoid excessive strain on the repair site. Early active extension and passive flexion are begun after 2 weeks, although weight bearing may be limited for 3 to 4 weeks.[41,46] Active plantar flexion and gentle-resistance strength training with elastic bands can be added after 8 weeks, advancing to toe raises and use of a stationary bike. Boot immobilization is discontinued around 8 to 10 weeks. Rehabilitation may be necessary for at least 3 to 4 months before patients resume jogging or dancing *en pointe*.

Although the literature on chronic FHL conditions is more expansive,[30,31,33,34,36–38] the literature on clinical outcomes after acute FHL tear is sparse, all consisting of level V case reports.[32,39–41,44,46] Although this limited group of patients had good relief of symptoms, return of strength, and resumption of exercise and dance activities, proper evidence-based recommendations remain poorly defined for this injury.

REFERENCES

1. Anouchi YS, Parker RD, Seitz WH. Posterior compartment syndrome of the calf resulting from misdiagnosis of a rupture of the medial head of the gastrocnemius. J Trauma 1987;27(6):678–80.
2. Froimson AI. Tennis leg. JAMA 1969;209(3):415–6.
3. Gilbert TJ, Bullis BR, Griffiths HJ. Tennis calf or tennis leg. Orthopedics 1996; 19(2):182–4.
4. Hoppenfeld S, deBoer P. Surgical exposures in orthopaedics: the anatomic approach. Edited. Philadelphia: J.B. Lippincott; 1994.
5. Garrett WE. Muscle strain injuries. Am J Sports Med 1996;24(6):S2–8.
6. Bianchi S, Martinoli C, Abdelwahab IF, et al. Sonographic evaluation of tears of the gastrocnemius medial head ("tennis leg"). J Ultrasound Med 1998;17:157–62.
7. Blue JM, Matthews LS. Leg injuries. Clin Sports Med 1997;16(3):467–78.
8. Clanton TO, Schon LC. Athletic inuries to the soft tissues of the foot and ankle. In: Mann R, Coughlin M, editors. Surgery of the foot and ankle. 6th edition. St. Louis (MO): Mosby; 1993. p. 1095–224.
9. Johnson EW. Tennis leg. Am J Phys Med Rehabil 2000;79(3):221.
10. Kwak H-S, Han Y-M, Lee S-Y, et al. Diagnosis and follow-up US evaluation of ruptures of the medial head of the gastrocnemius ("tennis leg"). Korean J Radiol 2006;7(3):193–8.
11. Kwak H-S, Lee K-B, Han Y-M. Ruptures of the medial head of the gastrocnemius ("tennis leg"): clinical outcome and compression effect. Clin Imaging 2006;30: 48–53.
12. Miller WA. Rupture of the musculotendinous juncture of the medial head of the gastrocnemius muscle. Am J Sports Med 1977;5(5):191–3.
13. Shields CL, Redix L, Brewster CE. Acute tears of the medial head of the gastrocnemius. Foot Ankle 1985;5(4):186–90.
14. Slawski DP. Deep venous thrombosis complicating rupture of the medial head of the gastrocnemius muscle. J Orthop Trauma 1994;8(3):263–4.
15. Touliopolous S, Hershman EB. Lower leg pain - diagnosis and treatment of compartment syndromes and other pain syndromes of the leg. Sports Med 1999;27(3):193–204.
16. Yilmaz C, Orgenc Y, Ergenc R, et al. Rupture of the medial gastrocnemius muscle during namaz praying: an unusual cause of tennis leg. Comput Med Imaging Graph 2008;32:728–31.
17. Zecher SB, Leach RE. Lower leg and foot injuries in tennis and other racquet sports. Clin Sports Med 1995;14(1):223–39.
18. Delgado GJ, Chung CB, Lektrakul N, et al. Tennis leg: clinical US study of 141 patients and anatomic investigation of four cadavers with MR imaging and US. Radiology 2002;224(1):112–9.
19. Ozcakar L, Solak HN, Yorubulut M. Letter to the editor. J Am Geriatr Soc 2005; 53(2):356–7.
20. Sando B. Calf strain. Aust Fam Physician 1988;17(12):1060–1.
21. Menz MJ, Lucas GL. Magnetic resonance imaging of a rupture of the medial head of the gastrocnemius muscle. J Bone Joint Surg Am 1991;73(8):1260–2.
22. Severance HW, Bassett FH. Rupture of the plantaris - does it exist? J Bone Joint Surg Am 1982;64(9):1387–8.
23. Hamilton W, Klostermeier T, Lim EV, et al. Surgically documented rupture of the plantaris muscle: a case report and literature review. Foot Ankle Int 1997;18(8): 522–3.

24. Helms CA, Fritz RC, Garvin GJ. Plantaris muscle injury: evaluation with MR imaging. Radiology 1995;195:201–3.
25. Cavalier R, Gabos PG, Bowen JR. Isolated rupture of the soleus muscle: a case report. Am J Orthop 1998;27:755–7.
26. Lopez GJ, Hoffman RS, Davenport M. Plantaris rupture: a mimic of deep venous thrombosis. J Emerg Med 2009 Jan 14 [Epub ahead of print].
27. Mennen U. Letter to the editor. J Bone Joint Surg Am 1983;65:1030.
28. Allard JC, Bancroft J, Porter G. Imaging of plantaris muscle rupture. Clin Imaging 1992;16(1):55–8.
29. Leekam RN, Agur AM, McKee NH. Using sonography to diagnose injury of plantaris muscles and tendons. AJR Am J Roentgenol 1999;172:185–9.
30. Hamilton WG. Stenosing tenosynovitis of the flexor hallucis longus tendon and posterior impingement upon the Os trigonum in ballet dancers. Foot Ankle 1982;3(2):74–80.
31. Hamilton WG, Geppert MJ, Thompson FM. Pain in the posterior aspect of the ankle in dancers: differential diagnosis and operative treatment. J Bone Joint Surg Am 1996;78(10):1491–500.
32. Inokuchi S, Usami N. Closed complete rupture of the flexor hallucis longus tendon at the groove of the talus. Foot Ankle Int 1997;18(1):47–9.
33. Kolettis GJ, Micheli LJ, Klein JD. Release of the flexor hallucis longus tendon in ballet dancers. J Bone Joint Surg Am 1996;78(9):1386–90.
34. Michelson J, Dunn L. Tenosynovitis of the flexor hallucis longus: a clinical study of the spectrum of presentation and treatment. Foot Ankle Int 2005;26(4):291–303.
35. Renard M, Simonet J, Boncteux P, et al. Intermittent dislocation of the flexor hallucis longus tendon. Skeletal Radiol 2003;32:78 81.
36. Sammarco GJ, Cooper PS. Flexor hallucis longus tendon injury in dancers and nondancers. Foot Ankle Int 1998;19(6):356–62.
37. Theodore GH, Kolettis GJ, Micheli LJ. Tenosynovitis of the flexor hallucis longus in a long-distance runner. Med Sci Sports Exerc 1996;28(3):277–9.
38. Tudisco C, Puddu G. Stenosing tenosynovitis of the flexor hallucis longus tendon in a classical ballet dancer: a case report. Am J Sports Med 1984;12(5):403–4.
39. Sammarco GJ, Miller EH. Partial rupture of the flexor hallucis longus tendon in classical ballet dancers. J Bone Joint Surg Am 1979;61(1):149–50.
40. Wei SY, Kneeland JB, Okereke E. Complete atraumatic rupture of the flexor hallucis longus tendon: a case report and review of the literature. Foot Ankle Int 1998;19:472–4.
41. Trepman E, Mizel MS, Newberg AH. Partial rupture of the flexor hallucis longus tendon in a tennis player: a case report. Foot Ankle Int 1995;16(4):227–31.
42. Krackow KA. Acute, traumatic rupture of a flexor hallucis longus tendon: a case report. Clin Orthop Rel Res 1980;150:261–2.
43. Coghlan BA, Clarke NMP. Traumatic rupture of the flexor hallucis longus tendon in a marathon runner. Am J Sports Med 1993;21(4):617–8.
44. Holt KW, Cross MJ. Isolated rupture of the flexor hallucis longus tendon: a case report. Am J Sports Med 1990;18(6):645–6.
45. Howard PD. Differential diagnosis of calf pain and weakness: flexor hallucis longus strain. J Orthop Sports Phys Ther 2000;30(2):78–84.
46. Thompson FM, Snow SW, Hershon SJ. Spontaneous atraumatic rupture of the flexor hallucis longus tendon under the sustentaculum tali: case report, review of the literature, and treatment options. Foot Ankle Int 1993;14(7):414–7.

Achilles Tendon Rehabilitation

Adam C. Strom[a], Mark M. Casillas, MD[b,c],*

KEYWORDS

- Achilles tendon • Rupture • Rehabilitation • Physical therapy
- Early mobilization • Late mobilization

The operative management of acute Achilles tendon rupture marks the beginning of a thoughtful, comprehensive and responsive rehabilitation program. The goals of the rehabilitation program start with the reduction of pain and swelling and progress toward the gradual recovery of ankle motion and power. Rehabilitation concludes with the restoration of coordinated activity and safe return to athletic activity.

Successfully rehabilitating a repaired acute Achilles tendon rupture requires a thorough understanding of the Achilles anatomy, injury, cellular repair mechanisms, and the patient's age, medical history, social history, and athletic activities. Taking these factors into consideration, an individualized Achilles rehabilitation protocol is prescribed for each patient. The protocol is considered dynamic and is modified as mandated by the clinical findings.

The length of immobilization and non–weight-bearing status during the rehabilitation period have long been discussed in the medical literature. Traditionally, immobilizing the ankle for the first few weeks after an Achilles injury was believed to allow adequate remodeling of the tendon, and stabilization of the wound. However, recent research suggests that early functional treatment with early weight-bearing and early motion results in statistically similar functional outcomes, allowing the patient to return to normal activity at a faster rate.[1–6]

ANATOMY, PHYSIOLOGY AND PATHOPHYSIOLOGY

The Achilles tendon forms at the junction of the medial and lateral gastrocnemius and soleus muscles. The medial and lateral gastrocnemius muscles originate on the posterior aspect of the medial and lateral femoral condyles, respectively. The soleus

[a] 3403 Hinman, Dartmouth College, Hanover, NH 03755, USA
[b] The Foot and Ankle Center of South Texas, 414 Navarro, Suite 1616, San Antonio, TX 78205, USA
[c] Department of Orthopedic Surgery, The University of Texas Health Science Center at San Antonio, TX 78229, USA
* Corresponding author. The Foot and Ankle Center of South Texas, 414 Navarro, Suite 1616, San Antonio, Texas 78205, USA
E-mail address: mmcasillas@satx.rr.com (M.M. Casillas).

Foot Ankle Clin N Am 14 (2009) 773–782
doi:10.1016/j.fcl.2009.08.003
1083-7515/09/$ – see front matter © 2009 Elsevier Inc. All rights reserved.

originates on the posterior tibia and fibula. The 3 muscles and their respective tendons contribute to the Achilles tendon, which in turn inserts into the posterior calcaneus. The Achilles tendon is surrounded by the paratenon, which is thinner than the synovial sheaths surrounding other tendons. The mesotenon, the middle layer of the paratenon, supplies most of the blood to the tendon, with the tendon also receiving blood from both the muscle or bone interfaces. Aström and Westlin note that blood flow is distributed evenly throughout the tendon, but is lower near the calcaneal insertion; during contraction, blood flow to the tendon is greatly diminished and can cease completely.[7]

With age, degradation of tendons occurs as a result of changes in the molecular properties of collagen, primarily caused by a low rate of regeneration and replacement, a reduction in the water content, and a decrease in vascular supply.[8] The degradation manifests as a weakening and stiffening of the Achilles tendon. Ippolito and colleagues,[9] in a histologic examination of rabbit tendons of varying ages, found increased bundling and density caused by increased collagen cross-linking in older specimens compared with the many individual and elastic fibers in young tendon. For the older, athletically active patient, these findings exemplify the need for a comprehensive stretching program with the intent of increasing the pliability of the Achilles tendon before strenuous loads are applied.

Complete rupture of the Achilles tendon can occur as the result of either chronic degeneration of the tendon, failure of the inhibitory mechanism of the musculotendinous unit, or direct or indirect trauma.[10,11] An area of decreased vascularity exists in the tendon, specifically at the region of insertion. It is well documented that with increasing age, blood flow at the extremities often diminishes, and regeneration is unable to occur at an adequate rate, resulting in a weakened tendon that is apt for complete rupture.[9,11,12] Mechanical failure can occur with either direct or indirect trauma caused by excessive loading, as might occur during the start of a sprint, or a sudden and violent plantarflexion or dorsiflexion of the ankle or foot that might occur during an unintentional step into a hole or a fall from a significant height.[10,11]

Acute rupture of the Achilles tendon can also occur on top of chronic overuse phenomena such as peritendinitis and tendinosis. Peritendinitis and tendinosis are the results of repetitive impact loading and microtrauma. These injuries can be caused intrinsically by decreased vascularity, aging, or anatomic deviation, or extrinsically by a change in athletic activity or exercise conditions.[10,12] Partial or complete Achilles rupture is a common finding during operative management, especially in athletes[7,10,13] These acute-on-chronic injuries are the result of degeneration in the tendon caused by tendinosis[11,14,15] and are suggested by Aström to result from degenerative microrupturing of collagen fibers.[16] Weakening of the tendon's cellular structure, as caused by peritendinitis and tendinosis, disposes the tendon to rupture during stress loads that would otherwise not result in any injury. The hypoxic degenerative lesions of peritendinitis and tendinosis are hypothesized to be a reason for increased blood flow in injured Achilles tendons.[17] A recent prospective study examined the microcirculation in limbs with insertional tendinopathy using power Doppler and concluded that microcirculatory blood flow is increased at the point of pain, whereas an asymptomatic limb showed no change in microcirculation.[13]

The 3 phases of tendon healing are similar to those of other soft tissue. The phases overlap to varying degrees. Immediately following injury, an inflammatory response occurs, supplying a source of cells for tendon repair. The inflammatory phase is followed by a period of new cell proliferation and increased vascularity while concurrently, collagen synthesis begins and the fibers enter a phase of maturation. Finally, a specific period of remodeling initiates as the newly formed collagen orients with the appropriate stresses for the region.

IMMOBILIZATION

For complete ruptures of the Achilles tendon, the mainstay of postoperative management is initial rigid immobilization in an equinus cast. The immobilization is followed by a supervised rehabilitation focused on recovery of motion and power. The duration and position of immobilization is believed to allow for progressive healing of the incision and rupture by reducing the mechanical sheer at the repair site. During the initial stage of healing when collagen fibers begin to form, pronounced tension through the tendon can ruin any healing progress and drastically extend the time needed for complete healing.

Immobilization in the equinus position is most favorable as it places less stress on the operative wound and repaired tendon. It is in this position that perfusion to the operative site is the least impeded.

Conversely, immobilization in a dorsiflexed position reduces the tendency to lose dorsiflexion during postoperative immobilization. Sorrenti[4] showed that postoperative casting in slight dorsiflexion improves calf recovery and ankle range of motion.

The accepted methods of immobilization for the Achilles tendon include casting and removable devices (cast boots). Casting has the advantage of custom fit, fixed positioning, and guaranteed patient compliance. These advantages are offset by the increased costs associated with casting materials, skilled personnel required for application, and of course, single use. Removable devices can also place the limb in a specific position; however, they cannot guarantee patient compliance. Such devices do allow for better hygiene and convenience as they can be removed for bathing and driving. In addition, these devices can be removed and adjusted at no additional cost to the patient.

Despite the significant benefits of postoperative immobilization, care must be given to avoid the well-documented detrimental effects of joint immobilization. These effects can include joint stiffness, muscle atrophy,[2,3,18,19] tendocutaneous adhesions,[3,18,19] deep vein thrombosis,[2,3,19] and ulceration of the joint cartilage.[2]

It is necessary to balance the detrimental effects with the time necessary for the tendon to successfully heal. Traditionally, 6 to 8 weeks has been the accepted length of immobilization.[3,18,20] More than this period, the amount of plantar flexion applied to the injured limb is gradually decreased in an attempt to increase dorsiflexion.

Significant debate exists in the literature regarding the appropriate length of post-surgical immobilization. Whereas past assumptions regarding the healing process and the correct length of rehabilitation have satisfactorily justified 6 to 8 weeks of non–weight-bearing status, recent, randomized, controlled studies suggest that early weight bearing does not impair recovery.[3,5,18,20] Specifically, early weight bearing is believed to decrease muscle atrophy and hasten the soft tissue healing process, including improved orientation of new collagen fibers.[21] Comparison between the studies is difficult because of differences in rehabilitation protocol.

Suchak[5] showed in a randomized study (n = 101) that early weight bearing resulted in similar recovery of strength in comparison to non–weight-bearing studies. Several patients were lost to follow-up, decreasing the statistical power of the results. The study remains 1 of the largest performed for early weight-bearing status of the Achilles. However, the randomized groups showed no appreciable difference in the rate of complications.

A study involving early motion by Mandelbaum and colleagues,[2] published in 1995 (n = 29), did not include a control group, and merely evaluated the outcomes of patients who underwent early range of motion exercises. Range of motion exercises began 72 hours after surgery, and the patients remained in removable posterior splints when not active. The group experienced a 94% recovery of pre-injury functionality after 6 months.

Kangas and colleagues[1] conducted a randomized study (n = 50) in 2003 that restricted 1 group of patients to plantarflexion using a bottomless cast and the remaining patients to full casts for 6 weeks (with weight-bearing status after 3 weeks) for both groups. The study found that calf strength was better in the early motion group, but the small sample size limits the results. Other outcome variables showed no significant difference.

Mortensen and colleagues,[3] in a controlled study (n = 71), used radiographic markers to compare the completeness of tendon healing in early motion and conventional rehabilitation groups. Neither group experienced increased lengthening of the tendon, and the early motion group experienced fewer tendocutaneous adhesions and an earlier return to work. The earlier return to work is correlated to an earlier increase in range of motion for the early weight-bearing group. Despite this early return of motion, both groups ultimately achieved the same range of motion. The investigators also noted no appreciable differences in calf atrophy.

It has also been suggested that even with nonoperative management, early weight bearing yields good results.[22]

An anatomic study by Stehno-Bittel and colleagues[18] confirms the benefits of early motion at the cellular level. The paper concludes that functional casting improves biochemical and biomechanical properties of the tendon. Evidence at the cellular level, in conjunction with the studies mentioned earlier, provides support for early mobilization during Achilles rupture rehabilitation.

None of the studies discussed earlier reported rates of complications, including re-rupture, that differ from the traditional treatment of immobilization. However, cross-study comparison was made difficult by the variety of repair methods used. Due to an associated faster functional recovery and more expedient return to work, several statistically powerful studies support early mobilization.

ADDITIONAL CONSIDERATIONS
Athletic Activity

For surgical management of tendinopathy, Maffulli and colleagues[23] write that nonathletic patients tend to experience a lengthened period of recovery, a higher rate of complications, and are at an increased risk for additional surgery. Athletic patients were defined as those exceeding an hour of physical activity each week. Of the 48 nonathletic patients, only 23 obtained normal levels of activity at the end of the study; it is speculated that the better outcome of athletic patients is influenced by their increased motivation, access to rehabilitation programs, and enhanced direction. Athletically inclined patients can undergo a more vigorous rehabilitation program, whereas more sedentary patients require a traditional approach.

Age

Aging also directly affects the patient's rehabilitation course as a result of changes at the cellular level. With increased age, there is notably increased collagen cross-linking. These new structures are realized in stiffness and an overall loss of elasticity in the Achilles tendon.[9,11,12] Older patients therefore require a less aggressive treatment protocol with special attention to warm-up and cool-down exercises.

Associated Medical Conditions

The patient's smoking status may compound the healing process and require adjustment of the rehabilitation program. The extrinsic effects of smoking can include the impedance of cutaneous blood flow.[24] At the cellular level, the effects of prolonged smoking can include decreased proliferation of red blood cells, fibroblasts, and macrophages, all key components of the wound healing process. Fibroblasts are needed for the scaffolding of collagen, and a sufficient level of oxygen must be supplied by red blood cells for healthy scar formation. Other chemicals present in cigarette smoke, such as hydrogen cyanide, can compound deficiencies in enzyme formation and oxygen transportation.[25]

It is also important to consider the patient's currently prescribed medications before establishing the treatment program. Specific consideration must be given to corticosteroids, as these drugs diminish the tensile strength of the Achilles. Animal studies have indicated that tissue necrosis occurs at the exact site of local steroid injection.[26] In addition to corticosteroids, fluoroquinolone antibiotics can also detrimentally affect tendon structure.[11,26]

Patients with systemic diseases such as rheumatoid arthritis and systemic lupus erythematosus require an extended rehabilitation period. Weakened collagen and degraded joint surfaces may inhibit the healing of the tendon.[11]

GOALS FOR REHABILITATION

Supervised rehabilitation provides a programmed course for daily Achilles rehabilitation directed to the completion of the specified goals (Table 1). The supervision allows for close monitoring of the repair, and provides positive feedback to the patient. The program is prescribed by the surgeon and administered by the surgeon or preferably by the athletic trainer or physical therapist. For patients with limited resources, the orthopedic surgeon can administer the rehabilitation program. The administration is time consuming but can be facilitated by handouts and instructions provided by the medical assistant or orthopedic technologist. The administration of the rehabilitation program through the orthopedic surgeon's office has the significant disadvantage of limited patient visits and is reliant on patient compliance.

The main advantage of a rehabilitation program administered by an athletic trainer or physical therapist is the increased number of patient contacts. Frequent visits provide a more complete clinical follow-up and increase the amount of feedback that is offered to the patient. Training errors can be quickly identified and corrected and the rehabilitation program itself can by modified to best accommodate the specific needs of the patient. The increased frequency of feedback motivates the patient to participate in the rehabilitation program and avoid restricted activities.

The first goal of the rehabilitation program is to address residual pain and swelling. Massage and ice are used to manage the residual pain. Massage, differential compression, graduated compression garment, ice, contrast baths, and electrical stimulation are useful adjuncts to manage the residual swelling.

The second goal of the rehabilitation program is to recover motion while preserving the integrity of the repair. The therapist or trainer must continuously assess the clinical

Table 1	
The goals of the acute Achilles tendon rupture postoperative rehabilitation program	
Goal 1	Reduce residual pain and swelling
Goal 2	Recover ankle dorsiflexion while protecting the repair
Goal 3	Safely strengthen the gastrocnemius-soleus-Achilles motor unit
Goal 4	Improve the strength and coordination of the entire lower extremity
Goal 5	Provide a safe and competitive return to athletic activity

findings to adjust the tension applied to the repair during the course of the rehabilitation program. Warm-up, including massage and deep heat modalities, is used in conjunction with stretching to recover dorsiflexion. The anatomy of the gastrocnemius-soleus-Achilles motor unit allows for isolated stretching of the gastrocnemius muscles and the soleus-Achilles (**Fig. 1**). The 2 stretches exploit the fact that the gastrocnemius inserts above the knee and the soleus originates exclusively on the tibia. Isolated gastrocnemius muscle stretch is accomplished with the knee extended, whereas isolated soleus-Achilles stretch is accomplished with the knee flexed.

In joints with stiff and contracted capsules, forced range of motion produces undesirable compressive forces across the joint surfaces. To address this problem, joint mobilization emphasizes joint distraction and translations before range of motion is attempted. Once the capsule is stretched and mobilized then range of motion is performed with a simultaneous joint distraction.

The third goal of the rehabilitation program is to safely strengthen the gastrocnemius-soleus-Achilles motor unit. The isolated strengthening of the motor unit is accomplished with a graduated program of resistance strengthening using elastic bands and closed-chain exercises. The closed-chain exercises maintain foot contact with the ground or device and are considered safer than open-chain activities that do not maintain foot contact. Examples of closed-chain activities in order of increasing difficulty include seated calf pumps, bipedal calf pumps, single leg calf pumps, and single leg calf pumps on a balance board or trampoline.

The fourth goal of the rehabilitation program is to improve the strength and coordination of the entire lower extremity. The concepts used in the isolated strengthening of the gastrocnemius-soleus-Achilles motor unit are also applied to the entire extremity. The rehabilitation is facilitated by the incorporation of swimming, water jogging, and the exercise cycling to the program.

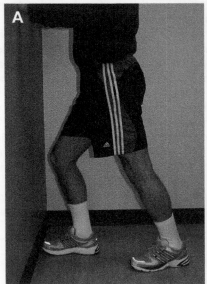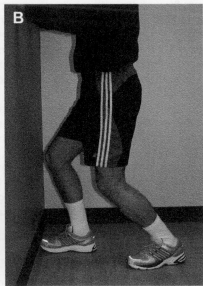

Fig. 1. Isolated stretching of the gastrocnemius muscles and the soleus-Achilles unit facilitates gastrocnemius-soleus-Achilles stretching. The 2 stretches exploit the fact that the gastrocnemius inserts above the knee, whereas the soleus originates exclusively on the tibia. (*A*) Isolated gastrocnemius muscle stretch with the knee extended. (*B*) Isolated soleus-Achilles stretch with the knee flexed.

The fifth goal of the rehabilitation program is to provide a safe and competitive return to athletic activity. The focus is on the avoidance of re-injury, namely, re-rupture of the Achilles tendon, while simultaneously rehabilitating the gastrocnemius-soleus-Achilles motor unit, the injured extremity, and the athlete. To accomplish this, the program incorporates cross training with cycle- and water-based activities to promote aerobic recovery while promoting coordinated motor activity in both lower extremities.

AUTHORS'ACUTE ACHILLES TENDON RUPTURE POSTOPERATIVE PROTOCOL

Our rehabilitation protocol for the repair of the acute Achilles tendon is driven by the clinical history, the operative findings, and the repair technique (**Table 2**). The protocol can be modified as necessary to maximize recovery and minimize complications. The period of immobilization is shortened by 1 to 2 weeks for athletic and compliant patients without other comorbidities. The initial 6-week non–weight-bearing period is typically left unaltered in an effort to reduce the risk for re-rupture.

In the most common case, the acute Achilles rupture is primarily repaired by re-approximation with nonabsorbable core sutures, a peripheral repair of the tendon with a smaller suture, followed by a complete closure of the paratenon. The ankle is immobilized in gravity equinous with a padded plaster splint.

Each postoperative visit provides the surgeon with an opportunity to identify superficial infection, deep infection, re-rupture, and deep vein thrombosis. To that end, each

Table 2	
Authors' acute Achilles tendon rupture postoperative protocol	
Day 1	Elevation Non-weight bearing Toe motion
Day 10	Suture removal Short leg cast with reduced equinous Non-weight bearing Toe motion
Day 17	Short leg cast with reduced equinous Non-weight bearing Toe motion
Day 24	Short leg cast with neutral ankle dorsiflexion Non-weight bearing Toe motion
Week 6	Removable cast boot (± night use) ± Night splint Weight bearing Physical therapy program: joint mobilization, stretching, strengthening Cross training
Week 9	Removable cast boot (± night use) ± Night splint Weight bearing Physical therapy program: proprioceptive and functional ankle recovery Cross training
Week 12	Discontinue cast boot Physical therapy program: return to sport phase, road running Cross training
Week 16	Release to full activity Emphasize stretching and warm-up

visit includes a review of systems that incorporates questions related to fever, chills, shortness of breath, chest pain, cough, calf pain, and incision pain. Each visit includes a measurement of the patient's temperature, and an inspection of the incision, and inspection and palpation of the Achilles repair and the calf with attention directed to draining, erythema, swelling, or defects at the repair site, and calf swelling or tenderness.

Day 1

The patient is instructed to keep the extremity at bed level or higher and to remain strictly non-weight bearing. Toe motion is encouraged.

Day 10

If the wound is sealed then the sutures are removed and a short leg cast is applied. The equinous ankle position is reduced slightly by casting the patient in the prone position while a qualified assistant carefully applies a slight dorsiflexion force. No attempt is made to correct to neutral ankle dorsiflexion. Strict non-weight bearing is maintained and toe motion encouraged.

Day 17

The first cast is removed and a short leg cast is re-applied with an additional gradual correction of the ankle equinous. Strict non-weight bearing is maintained and toe motion encouraged.

Day 24

The second cast is removed and a short leg cast is re-applied with complete correction of the ankle equinous. If the Achilles remains tight then allow ample time for gentle stretching and include massage of the gastrocnemius to facilitate lengthening before cast application. Strict non-weight bearing is maintained and toe motion encouraged.

Week 6

The third cast is removed and a removable cast boot is applied. The boot is used day and night. Alternatively, a night splint is used to provide passive dorsiflexion stretch. The patient is placed in a physical therapy program and allowed to start weight bearing.

The physical therapy program is directed toward recovery of motion and power. Pain and swelling are not typically problematic at this stage. Each session starts with application of moist heat, gentle leg massage, and gentle stretching. If joint stiffness is pronounced then ankle and subtalar joint mobilization is performed in addition to simple range of motion. The gastrocnemius and soleus-Achilles are stretched in isolation as outlined earlier. As the motion is recovered and the repair matures stretching becomes more intensive and strengthening is addressed. Initially, coordinated motion with toe alphabets is followed by the addition of elastic band concentric exercises. Resistance is gradually increased and eccentric and closed-chain exercises are added.

Cross training for aerobic conditioning includes swimming, aqua jogging, and exercise cycling. In additional, upper extremity weight training, limited lower extremity weight training, and core strengthening are used for conditioning.

Week 9

The patient is kept in a removable cast boot for daily activities. The use of the boot or splint at night is discontinued unless range of motion remains limited. Progress with physical therapy is assessed and the program is fine-tuned. Typically, the program is advanced to full proprioceptive and functional ankle recovery with the addition of uneven boards and small trampolines.

Week 12

The cast boot is discontinued and used on an as-needed basis. The physical therapy program is shifted to a return to sport phase. Plyometrics, sport-specific drills, and the progressive use of the elliptical trainer, treadmill, and road running are added to the program.

Week 16

The final assessment verifies that the tendon is not tender and that the ankle has recovered full dorsiflexion. The patient is released to full activity with an emphasis on stretching and warm-up.

The protocol must be modified to accommodate complications. The possibility of superficial infection demands more frequent visits, immobilization, and oral antibiotics. The possibility of a deep infection demands appropriate workup, antibiotics, and surgical debridement.

At the sixth week, the ankle should be at neutral dorsiflexion. More frequent and progressively more aggressive cast changes can be used in the first 6 weeks following Achilles repair. During the second 6-week period the ankle should dorsiflex to progressively greater degrees above neutral. If the progress is slow then add a dorsiflexion night splint or a dorsiflexion-assist ankle foot orthosis. The physical therapist must be reasonably aggressive given the specific surgical and clinical findings.

Persistent Achilles pain is a difficult problem. The authors aggressively reverse the rehabilitation course and place patients back in cast. For less dramatic cases the patient is placed back into a boot and night splint, and the physical therapy modified to include more modalities such as ultrasound and electrical stimulation. For recalcitrant cases the authors use a solid ankle foot orthosis in an effort to keep the patient as mobile and comfortable as possible. We are quick to obtain laboratory work to rule out occult infection and magnetic resonance imaging to assess the repair site. Occasionally, removal of the core suture is performed in an effort to reduce Achilles pain associated with possible strangulation of tendon fibers.

REFERENCES

1. Kangas J, Pajala A, Siira P, et al. Early functional treatment versus early immobilization in tension of the musculotendinous unit after Achilles rupture repair: a prospective, randomized, clinical study. J Trauma 2003;54:1171–81.
2. Mandelbaum BR, Myerson MS, Forster R. Achilles tendon ruptures. A new method of repair, early range of motion, and functional rehabilitation. Am J Sports Med 1995;23:392–5.
3. Mortensen HM, Skov O, Jensen PE. Early motion of the ankle after operative treatment of a rupture of the Achilles tendon. A prospective, randomized clinical and radiographic study. J Bone Joint Surg Am 1999;81:983–90.
4. Sorrenti SJ. Achilles tendon rupture: effect of early mobilization in rehabilitation after surgical repair. Foot Ankle Int 2006;27:407–10.
5. Suchak AA, Bostick GP, Beaupre LA, et al. The influence of early weight-bearing compared with non-weight-bearing after surgical repair of the Achilles tendon. J Bone Joint Surg Am 2008;90:1876–83.

6. Twaddle BC, Poon P. Early motion for Achilles tendon ruptures: is surgery important? A randomized, prospective study. Am J Sports Med 2007;35:2033–8.
7. Astrom M, Westlin N. Blood flow in chronic Achilles tendinopathy. Clin Orthop Relat Res 1994;308:166–72.
8. Fischgrund JS, American Academy of Orthopaedic Surgeons. OKU 9: orthopaedic knowledge update. Rosemont,(IL): American Academy of Orthopaedic Surgeons; 2008.
9. Ippolito E, Natali PG, Postacchini F, et al. Morphological, immunochemical, and biochemical study of rabbit Achilles tendon at various ages. J Bone Joint Surg Am 1980;62:583–98.
10. DeLee J, Drez D, Miller MD, et al. DeLee & Drez's orthopaedic sports medicine. 2nd edition. Philadelphia: Saunders; 2003.
11. Leppilahti J, Orava S. Total Achilles tendon rupture: a review. Sports Med 1998; 25:79–100.
12. Kannus P, Paavola M, Paakkala T, et al. Pathophysiology of overuse tendon injury. Radiologe 2002;42:766–70.
13. Knobloch K, Kraemer R, Lichtenberg A, et al. Achilles tendon and paratendon microcirculation in midportion and insertional tendinopathy in athletes. Am J Sports Med 2006;34:92.
14. Schepsis AA, Jones H, Haas AL. Achilles tendon disorders in athletes. Am J Sports Med 2002;30:287–305.
15. Skeoch DU. Spontaneous partial subcutaneous ruptures of the tendo achillis: review of the literature and evaluation of 16 involved tendons. Am J Sports Med 1981;9:20.
16. Åström M. Partial rupture in chronic Achilles tendinopathy: a retrospective analysis of 342 cases. Acta Orthop 1998;69:404–7.
17. Zanetti M, Metzdorf A, Kundert HP, et al. Achilles tendons: clinical relevance of neo-vascularization diagnosed with power Doppler US. Radiology 2003;227:556–60.
18. Stehno-Bittel L, Reddy GK, Gum S, et al. Biochemistry and biomechanics of healing tendon: part I. Effects of rigid plaster casts and functional casts. Med Sci Sports Exerc 1998;30:788–93.
19. Troop RL, Losse GM, Lane JG, et al. Early motion after repair of Achilles tendon ruptures. Foot Ankle Int 1995;16:705–9.
20. Wills CA, Washburn S, Caiozzo V, et al. Achilles tendon rupture. A review of the literature comparing surgical versus nonsurgical treatment. Clin Orthop Relat Res 1986;207:156–63.
21. Gelberman RH, Menon J, Gonsalves M, et al. The effects of mobilization on the vascularization of healing flexor tendons in dogs. Section III. Clin Orthop Relat Res 1980;153:283–9.
22. Twaddle BC, Poon P, Monnig J. Randomised prospective study of surgical vs. non-surgical treatment of Achilles tendon rupture-clinical results [abstract]. J Bone Joint Surg Br 2005;87:30.
23. Maffulli N, Testa V, Capasso G, et al. Surgery for chronic Achilles tendinopathy yields worse results in nonathletic patients. Clin J Sport Med 2006;16:123–8.
24. Leow YH, Maibach HI. Cigarette smoking, cutaneous vasculature, and tissue oxygen. Clin Dermatol 1998;16:579–84.
25. Silverstein P. Smoking and wound healing. Am J Med 1992;93:22S–4S.
26. Hugate R, Pennypacker J, Saunders M, et al. The effects of intratendinous and retrocalcaneal intrabursal injections of corticosteroid on the biomechanical properties of rabbit Achilles tendons. J Bone Joint Surg Am 2004;86-A:794–801.

Index

Note: Page numbers of article titles are in **boldface** type.

Foot Ankle Clin N Am 14 (2009) 783–804
doi:10.1016/S1083-7515(09)00090-4
1083-7515/09/$ – see front matter © 2009 Elsevier Inc. All rights reserved.

foot.theclinics.com

Moving?

Make sure your subscription moves with you!

To notify us of your new address, find your **Clinics Account Number** (located on your mailing label above your name), and contact customer service at:

Email: journalscustomerservice-usa@elsevier.com

800-654-2452 (subscribers in the U.S. & Canada)
314-447-8871 (subscribers outside of the U.S. & Canada)

Fax number: 314-447-8029

Elsevier Health Sciences Division
Subscription Customer Service
3251 Riverport Lane
Maryland Heights, MO 63043

1. Publication Title	2. Publication Number	3. Filing Date
Foot and Ankle Clinics	0 1 6 - 3 6 8	9/15/09

4. Issue Frequency	5. Number of Issues Published Annually	6. Annual Subscription Price
Mar, Jun, Sep, Dec	4	$230.00

7. Complete Mailing Address of Known Office of Publication (Not printer) (Street, city, county, state, and ZIP+4®)

Elsevier Inc.
360 Park Avenue South
New York, NY 10010-1710

Contact Person
Stephen Bushing

Telephone (Include area code)
215-239-3688

8. Complete Mailing Address of Headquarters or General Business Office of Publisher (Not printer)

Elsevier Inc., 360 Park Avenue South, New York, NY 10010-1710

9. Full Names and Complete Mailing Addresses of Publisher, Editor, and Managing Editor (Do not leave blank)

Publisher (Name and complete mailing address)

John Schrefer, Elsevier, Inc., 1600 John F. Kennedy Blvd. Suite 1800, Philadelphia, PA 19103-2899

Editor (Name and complete mailing address)

Deb Dellapena, Elsevier, Inc., 1600 John F. Kennedy Blvd. Suite 1800, Philadelphia, PA 19103-2899

Managing Editor (Name and complete mailing address)

Catherine Bewick, Elsevier, Inc., 1600 John F. Kennedy Blvd. Suite 1800, Philadelphia, PA 19103-2899

10. Owner (Do not leave blank. If the publication is owned by a corporation, give the name and address of the corporation immediately followed by the names and addresses of all stockholders owning or holding 1 percent or more of the total amount of stock. If not owned by a corporation, give the names and addresses of the individual owners. If owned by a partnership or other unincorporated firm, give its name and address as well as those of each individual owner. If the publication is published by a nonprofit organization, give its name and address.)

Full Name	Complete Mailing Address
Wholly owned subsidiary of	4520 East-West Highway
Reed/Elsevier, US holdings	Bethesda, MD 20814

11. Known Bondholders, Mortgagees, and Other Security Holders Owning or Holding 1 Percent or More of Total Amount of Bonds, Mortgages, or Other Securities. If none, check box ☐ None

Full Name	Complete Mailing Address
N/A	

12. Tax Status (For completion by nonprofit organizations authorized to mail at nonprofit rates) (Check one)
The purpose, function, and nonprofit status of this organization and the exempt status for federal income tax purposes:
☐ Has Not Changed During Preceding 12 Months
☐ Has Changed During Preceding 12 Months (Publisher must submit explanation of change with this statement)

PS Form 3526, September 2007 (Page 1 of 3 (Instructions Page 3)) PSN 7530-01-000-9931 PRIVACY NOTICE: See our Privacy policy in www.usps.com

13. Publication Title	14. Issue Date for Circulation Data Below
Foot and Ankle Clinics	June 2009

15. Extent and Nature of Circulation		Average No. Copies Each Issue During Preceding 12 Months	No. Copies of Single Issue Published Nearest to Filing Date
a. Total Number of Copies (Net press run)		1525	1500
b. Paid Circulation (By Mail and Outside the Mail)	(1) Mailed Outside-County Paid Subscriptions Stated on PS Form 3541. (Include paid distribution above nominal rate, advertiser's proof copies, and exchange copies)	846	808
	(2) Mailed In-County Paid Subscriptions Stated on PS Form 3541 (Include paid distribution above nominal rate, advertiser's proof copies, and exchange copies)		
	(3) Paid Distribution Outside the Mails Including Sales Through Dealers and Carriers, Street Vendors, Counter Sales, and Other Paid Distribution Outside USPS®	179	170
	(4) Paid Distribution by Other Classes Mailed Through the USPS (e.g. First-Class Mail®)		
c. Total Paid Distribution (Sum of 15b (1), (2), (3), and (4))	▶	1025	978
d. Free or Nominal Rate Distribution (By Mail and Outside the Mail)	(1) Free or Nominal Rate Outside-County Copies Included on PS Form 3541	85	80
	(2) Free or Nominal Rate In-County Copies Included on PS Form 3541		
	(3) Free or Nominal Rate Copies Mailed at Other Classes Through the USPS (e.g. First-Class Mail)		
	(4) Free or Nominal Rate Distribution Outside the Mail (Carriers or other means)		
e. Total Free or Nominal Rate Distribution (Sum of 15d (1), (2), (3) and (4))	▶	85	80
f. Total Distribution (Sum of 15c and 15e)	▶	1110	1058
g. Copies not Distributed (See instructions to publishers #4 (page #3))	▶	415	442
h. Total (Sum of 15f and g)	▶	1525	1500
i. Percent Paid (15c divided by 15f times 100)		92.34%	92.44%

16. Publication of Statement of Ownership

☐ If the publication is a general publication, publication of this statement is required. Will be printed in the December 2009 issue of this publication.

Publication not required

17. Signature and Title of Editor, Publisher, Business Manager, or Owner

Stephen R. Bushing

Stephen R. Bushing Subscription Service Coordinator

Date
September 15, 2009

I certify that all information furnished on this form is true and complete. I understand that anyone who furnishes false or misleading information on this form or who omits material or information requested on the form may be subject to criminal sanctions (including fines and imprisonment) and/or civil sanctions (including civil penalties).

PS Form 3526, September 2007 (Page 2 of 3)

Printed and bound by CPI Group (UK) Ltd, Croydon, CR0 4YY

03/10/2024

01040465-0020